SEARCHING FOR
slippers

one mom's coming of age story

By Stacy Ross

inspired **girl**

SEARCHING FOR SLIPPERS by Stacy Ross

Published by Inspired Girl, an imprint of Inspired Girl Publishing Group, a division of Inspired Girl Enterprises
Asbury Park, NJ 07712
inspiredgirlbooks.com

Inspired Girl Publishing Group is honored to bring forth books with heart and stories that matter. We are proud to offer this book to our readers; the story, the experiences, and the words are the author's alone.

The stories portrayed within *Searching for Slippers* are based on actual events. In some incidents, characteristics, names, and timelines may have been compressed or combined to protect the privacy and preserve the anonymity of people involved. The conversations in the book all come from the author's recollections, though they are not written to represent word-for-word transcripts.

This book is written as a source of information only. The information contained in this book should by no means be considered a substitute for the advice of a qualified medical professional. In addition, the publisher and the author assume no responsibility for errors, inaccuracies, omissions, or any other inconsistencies herein. The use of this book implies your acceptance of this disclaimer. Products, books, trademarks, and trademark names are used throughout this book to describe and inform the reader about various proprietary products that are owned by third parties. No endorsement of the information contained in this book is given by the owners of such products and trademarks, and no endorsement is implied by the inclusion of products, books, or trademarks in this book.

© 2025 Stacy Ross
All rights reserved. No portion of this book may be reproduced in any form without permission from the publisher, except as permitted by U.S. copyright law. For permissions: help@inspiredgirlbooks.com

ISBN Paperback: 978-1-965240-09-0
ISBN Hardcover: 978-1-965240-10-6
Written by: Stacy Ross
Editorial & Creative Director: Jenn Tuma-Young
Lead Editor: Natalie Papailiou
Proofreader: Briana Hall
Book Production: Inspired Girl Publishing Group
Library of Congress Control Number: 2024926557

This book is dedicated to my family, Howard, Leo, Emily, and Fin. I am so grateful to all of you for allowing me to share our story. It is because of you I still believe in fairytales.

"I wanted a perfect ending. Now I've learned the hard way that some poems don't rhyme, and some stories don't have a clear beginning, middle, and end. Life is about not knowing, having to change, taking the moment, and making the best of it, without knowing what's going to happen next."

- GILDA RADNOR

TABLE OF CONTENTS

NOTE TO READERS 09

PROLOGUE 11

CHAPTER ONE
Once Upon a Time. 19

CHAPTER TWO
Shake, Rattle, and Roll 25

CHAPTER THREE
And Baby Makes Three 33

CHAPTER FOUR
Finding Mrs. Fix-It 47

CHAPTER FIVE
A Fork in the Road 59

CHAPTER SIX
Warrior One 83

CHAPTER SEVEN
A Lot on the Line 95

CHAPTER EIGHT
When I Can't Talk, I Type 111

CHAPTER NINE
Therapy. Therapy. and More Therapy. 119

CHAPTER TEN
It's Not Easy Being Married to Superman. 133

CHAPTER ELEVEN
A Picture Is Worth a Thousand Words and a Transfer . . . 145

CHAPTER TWELVE
The Jury Is Out. 157

CHAPTER THIRTEEN
Transitions 175

CHAPTER FOURTEEN
A Soft Landing. 201

EPILOGUE 219

THROUGH FIN'S EYES 223

ACKNOWLEDGMENTS 227

CONTENT ADVISORY BOX

This book delves into mental health challenges, portraying characters navigating psychological struggles. It also explores aspects of psychology and mental health and contains depictions of self-harm, bullying, hospitalization, and suicide ideation. This book also contains themes of infertility. Please read with care.

NOTE TO READERS

As I set out to tell my story, I knew that it would be difficult, and I would be tempted to gloss over some of the things that I'm less than proud of, or even omit things I wish I did differently. But I felt the only way to truly show who I've become was to be unwaveringly honest about where I've been. I am only able to share the most vulnerable times in my life because I know at each turn I made the best decision I could with what I knew at the time, and I kept growing. It is also why I chose to share some of the lighter moments. I hope you will recognize yourself in both. As you read, please understand these are snapshots of my life chosen carefully to put together a full picture.

- *Stacy*

PROLOGUE

"911. What's your emergency?"

"It's my daughter. She broke a window. I'm worried she's a danger to herself and possibly us."

Our voices both so matter of fact, it seemed more likely we were starting a DoorDash order then a rescue mission. I realized how numb I had become in these situations.

We were having an early dinner. Grabbing some last moments together before we scattered to celebrate the New Year. The Chinese food containers passed as quickly around the table as our conversation changed topics. I don't remember exactly what triggered Molly, but I will never forget what followed.

It was like a switch being thrown. The light went out in her eyes, and she became almost predator-like. Ferocious in her words and uncontrolled in her motions, she glared around the table at her brother, her sister, my husband Howie, and me, deciding who she would pounce on next.

We sat at the round dining room table like animals at a standoff. Taking turns confronting our attacker in the hopes she would back down.

Our attacker was Molly's brain, registering us and whatever triggered her as a threat. It was her mental illness—borderline personality disorder—that took over our sweet, blonde-haired, blue-eyed girl with the giggle that could get everyone around her laughing.

I wanted that little girl to see me through whatever it was that was invading her mind. I tried to find that younger version of Molly whenever things got out of control. I knew she was in there, buried in the sixteen-year-old stranger staring me down from across the table. I went first, in as calm a voice as I could muster.

"Molly, this is silly; we have a fun night ahead of us. Everyone is coming over to celebrate New Year's. Let's just start over."

Sometimes the offer of letting her start over gave the disease a way out and quieted things down. Not tonight.

I tried so many times to fix her. I saw this coming. I wanted to fix her before it grew into this. Get her help or meds or whatever she needed. Damn those teachers who told me she was fine. Damn the misdiagnoses, one after the next. Damn the hospital stays that ended too soon before the fixing could happen, or the answers could be found.

Damn me. The mom who wanted everything picture-perfect and instead ended up with a literal shit show.

Did I do something to deserve this? Was this my karma for wanting the fairytale? The thoughts kept bubbling over like a pot of soup that's spent way too much time on the stovetop.

"No, Mother, we cannot just start over this time." Molly pounded the table with her fists and threw an open carton of lo mein at no one in particular. The carton hit the table with the full force of her anger, releasing the pungent smell of soy sauce and noodles into the air.

No one moved to clean it up.

Emily, ever the peacemaker, went next.

"Come on Molly, no one meant to upset you…" she pleaded with her big sister, hoping she would come back to us.

"Shut up, Emily, what do you know? You are one of Mom and Dad's perfect children who do nothing wrong. You just bring home perfect grades, perfect friends, perfect—"

She spat the words out as Emily visibly shrank back into her seat, scrunching up her face as tears started to stream down her cheeks.

"Molly, stop! You're just making things worse, and you don't mean it!" Emily's twin, Leo, yelled, always rooting for the good in everyone and acutely aware that this mental illness wasn't the fault of his big sister whom it was consuming. He was trying desperately to get her attention and stop the escalation.

I turned to Howie, quiet in his seat, observing. It was maddening that he sat there and allowed this to happen, but the look of incredulity on his face spoke volumes. On most days with him, it's like being married to Superman. But these situations were his kryptonite, and he sat there frozen like a deer in headlights.

I felt so alone. I couldn't understand why he just sat there, seemingly uninvolved, and let this escalate around him. The rage ignited by Molly boiled up inside me until it exploded sarcastically at Howie.

"Step in anytime."

Molly jumped at the opportunity to split us, pit us against one another.

"He's an idiot, Mom. He doesn't know what to say, and I won't acknowledge him."

The insults continued to fly from her mouth, so strong that her spit covered our open take-out cartons. It didn't matter, our appetites were gone. I couldn't help but think of the ten people who were due at our house in an hour.

Should I call them? Will she once again control and ultimately ruin an event? Change this New Year's memory into one that will always stand out?

I could not comprehend what was happening. Every time this happens, I am still in the same amount of disbelief. One minute, Molly is with us. The next she is gone, and we are all victims towing the line to her mental illness.

Howie and I told Leo and Emily they could leave the table. It was not a dismissal, and they did not see it that way. It was actually a welcome reprieve from what was going on. They were teenagers and had already turned the corner, becoming more protective of us in these situations. We tried to spare them from what we thought was pure abuse. We didn't try to shield them anymore—our house was by no means big enough to hide what was going on. We merely moved them out of the direct line of fire. They took the chance and went into the living room.

"Of course, excuse them! The perfect ones. If it wasn't for me, you'd have your perfect family, Mother. Boy, did you mess up. I'm sure you wish every day you didn't adopt me!" With every word, she pounded her fist on the dining room table, the already spilled lo mein bouncing up and down as if nodding along in agreement. Her teeth were clenching, and her eyes were squinting. The pain in her head seemed to be escaping like fire through her mouth.

She got angrier and angrier. No amount of discussion would soothe her. So, we sent her to her room as I tried to get some semblance of control and order back.

Even that was a fight, and she carried her anger upstairs like a wrecking ball. Every step up she stomped louder and louder, beating on the floors and rattling the house.

Suddenly we heard a crash, then glass shattering. We ran upstairs without thinking, stopping for a deep breath before throwing the door open. It was freezing. The December air blew in a freshly broken window.

Most disturbing was the pleased look in Molly's eyes.

I spoke. Slowly. With a control I did not even know I had. I stared right at her barely feeling the cold.

"Get in the car. You need to go to the hospital."

She refused. Backing away toward the open window. Her hands were trembling, as if she knew this wasn't her, but she couldn't control whatever it was. Howie dove and grabbed her. It was chilling to watch, the air feeling much colder than any open window could cause.

Without another thought, I walked downstairs and called the police.

To this day, I'm not sure if I did it because I was really scared or if I was following a script.

Child breaks window, threatens to hurt herself and you, becomes impossible to control. Call for help.

"911, What's your emergency?"

——— ,, ———

*Life is what
happens when you're
busy making plans.*

-JOHN LENNON

PART ONE

The Search is Over?

—— CHAPTER ONE ——

Once Upon a Time...

"We'll have one scoop of vanilla and one scoop of chocolate with Reese's Pieces and hot fudge," he ordered.

"Lots of Reese's Pieces and chocolate sprinkles too!" I added from the table for two I had staked out.

"Oh yes," he smiled, "how could I forget your chocolate sprinkles?"

Our easy banter was contagious and our classmate behind the counter laughed as he handed over our ice cream well hidden beneath a generous portion of toppings. Just the way I like it!

To anyone watching, it was obvious this wasn't our first date, and they would be right. We had been dating for almost four years and had shared many ice creams seated in the front window of Scoops, Collegetown's iconic ice cream shoppe. Tonight, however, was different. We had a big decision to make. One that could alter the course of our lives.

As much as we hated the idea, our time on the Hill was coming to a close. In just a few short weeks we would don our caps and gowns and march onto Schoellkopf Field with our 5,000+ classmates to collect our diplomas. Our paths, which led us to upstate New York four years ago, were now taking us in as many different directions. Many were heading to graduate school; law school seemed the most in vogue, probably attributed to the cult-like popularity of *LA Law*. Others, like me, were entertaining job offers that began with on-campus interviews and ended with promises of training programs and opportunities guaranteed to make the transition to a forty-hour work week, with only two weeks' vacation, painless.

While there were lots of senior couples, I believed that we were one of the few even considering making joint career decisions. We had spoken about a future together many times, but we had never fully considered the implications of including each other's career plans in our own. Like bell bottoms and leisure suits, it just wasn't in style.

Yet here we were. He was accepted into medical school in Rochester, New York, and waitlisted in several others in New York City. He could be accepted from the waitlist as late as August for a September start. I had job offers in both cities. As a product manager for a home product company in New York City and as an assistant buyer for a retail chain in Rochester. Both jobs had asked for an answer by May 1st.

As we took turns digging in, we talked about everything but why we came. Plans for the weekend, our last sorority and fraternity events, even finals. Anything to put off the inevitable. Too quickly, our spoons scraped the bottom and came to rest together in the empty sundae glass. We paused and took a breath, neither of us sure how to proceed. The size of the decision seemed too big for us, like we were playing a childhood game of dress-up. But, for what seemed the first time, the adult clothes fit, and it was time to step into our roles.

"Which job do you really want?" he began.

"Which school do you want to go to?" I answered.

Two questions, no answers. But we had broken the seal, and from there we kept talking. We laid out all the options. We analyzed the choices and attached probabilities to every scenario. We rationalized, we listed pros and cons, and we even discussed plan Bs.

Then everything changed. I don't remember how it started or who said it first, but the question we had been asking all along, *What is best for both of us?* became, *What would make us happiest?*

Suddenly being together became the only thing on the table. The mood lightened, and the rest was easy. A few formalities and a call to a Rochester rental agency made it official.

Howie and Stacy. College sweethearts. Met the first week, engaged the last. It was the fairytale I'd been writing, dreaming of, and expecting since childhood. Nothing so far had made me believe in anything else.

By today's standards, I led what would be described as a *privileged childhood*. My biggest concerns, bad acne and frizzy hair, were easily counteracted by two loving parents, a younger brother, a dog named Daisy, and grandparents who lived around the corner—not to mention a never-ending supply of Stridex pads and a good hair dryer!

School itself came pretty easy to me. A four-year member of the cheerleading squad, prom committee co-chair, and many other activities kept me busy and out of any real trouble. I graduated fifth in my class and was accepted into Cornell in February of my senior year. My family's faces at graduation when I looked up into the bleachers made it all worthwhile.

Howie and I met the first day of college in the U-Hall dorms common area, affectionately called *The Dustbowl*. I was homesick, and he was the perfect cure. At 6'1" with a build clearly giving away his obsession with body building, he could have been intimidating. However, his impish smile framed by Greg Bradyish curly brown hair, a t-shirt that ironically read *Kiss Me I'm Italian,* and lanky legs sticking far out of his corduroy OP shorts, made him warm and inviting. Howie was as dedicated to his studies as I was to having fun. He was pre-med; I wanted to do *something in communications.* He signed his love letters *H. Ross*, MD. I was hooked. For the next four years, we were inseparable.

From the beginning, Howie made me feel safe. When wrapped around me, his Popeye-sized arms seemed impenetrable. There wasn't much to protect me from back then except not having a date for a sorority date night. The up close and personal dating scene of the 80s was not for me. Today when I get together with my college roommates and listen to them reminisce about dates gone bad, and search for long lost boyfriends on social media, I'd still choose Howie every time.

I knew Howie was the one by spring of our junior year when I studied abroad in London with my roommate, Gail, while Howie prepared for the Medical School Boards *(MCATS)* back on campus. For four months we sent snail mail letters and cassette tapes across the Atlantic professing our love for each other.

By senior year, the butterflies were as strong as ever, and even though we began discussing a future together, my memories of that time are far from heavy. On one of the weekends just before our last set of finals, I left to visit my high school friend, Fredda, at University of Albany. I raced back in my '81 Corolla to meet Howie for dinner, singing at the top of my lungs to a playlist he made me.

I couldn't wait to see him. I knew he had an event at his fraternity house, so I started unpacking while I waited. It wasn't long before I heard a banging on the door.

"I'll get it," I yelled to Gail as I sprinted to the front door.

I'm not sure what struck me first. The smell of alcohol or the clothes Howie was wearing.

Then it hit me.

As I gazed at my boyfriend, dressed in only an extra small red blazer and corduroy shorts, I realized his zipper was open and it was painfully obvious to me, and to anyone who had seen him stumbling across campus, he was not wearing underwear.

All thoughts of a romantic homecoming gone; I slammed the door in his face.

He banged on the door again, apologizing and begging to be let in.

"Let the poor guy in, Stace. He already embarrassed himself enough for one night," Gail urged, giggling.

I couldn't stay mad at Howie. I opened the door again to him fumbling frantically with the zipper on his shorts and pulled him into the apartment while simultaneously pushing him away as he tried to hug me. He kept slurring, "Don't judge me, just love me," and I couldn't help but do just that.

Howie asked me to marry him the next week in a parking garage in downtown Ithaca after leaving my father a message on their answering machine and putting our favorite James Taylor song on in the car. Maybe not as extravagant or suave as the proposals of today, but it was romantic in its innocence. We celebrated that evening in our favorite Collegetown bar surrounded by our friends, and with our families the next week at graduation.

Two years later, I married my college sweetheart in what could only be described as a fairytale wedding. It was a rainy Saturday night in July; the ceremony called for 8:45 p.m. as our traditions made us wait until sundown. Even the rain was magical, casting an enchanting, mist-filled summer backdrop over the black and white themed ballroom. I believed the rain was good luck since both my parents and grandparents, married twenty-five and fifty years respectively at the time, told stories of their own shower-filled nuptials.

I remember taking a moment to myself at our table for two to look around the reception and take it all in. Everyone I loved was together in one room. Before I got too lost in my thoughts, the band's rendition of Sinatra's "New York, New York" brought me back to the party and onto the dancefloor. Just about every guest under twenty-five formed a kick line for the chorus, arms wrapped around each other, laughing with not a care in the world. That scene remains as vivid today as any photograph in our album. We were connected by more than our linked arms that day. Every one of us was filled with dreams of our own and blissfully unaware of what life had in store.

We were no different. We figured Howie would finish medical school and I would complete business school, getting a fabulous job in whatever city he did his residency and ultimately practiced in. We would have two to three children whenever we were ready and live somewhere in the Northeast, maintaining every friendship we treasured. It seemed so reasonable back then…plans turning into delicious reality with as much ease as a recipe tasting exactly like its mouthwatering picture.

CHAPTER TWO

Shake, Rattle, and Roll

"You want to have a baby?"
Howie looked down at me and smiled playfully.
"Like, now?"
"No, I'm serious. If we get pregnant now, we'll have the baby in New York with all our family and friends around!"

I was snuggled in close to Howie on our worn, brown couch in our first house, a 1967 split in West Hartford, CT. The TV was on, the Giants beating the Redskins in the 2nd quarter. It was a cold October afternoon and at 5:00 p.m. the sun was already lying low enough to stream in through the small casement window at the top of the wall. It felt homey, peaceful. I let a small smile curl at my lips as I pretended to be interested in the game.

As we sat in comfortable silence, allowing the life changing suggestion to sink in, I looked around. Our TV room was just four short steps down from the main level of our house. Long and narrow, this room ran the whole length of the house from front to back but was only about twelve feet wide. While we had furnished the front end with the couch and a 41" RCA TV, the part of the room toward the back of the house was empty. It would be the perfect play area for any child.

Howie was only two years into his surgical residency, and I was working as a Marketing Manager for BJ's Wholesale Club. Our combined income barely paid the bills and didn't even touch the medical school loans we deferred month after month. Howie had such a long road ahead of him that waiting for the *right time* was never going to come.

We drove to the White Mountains the next weekend for a romantic getaway. I was so sure I was pregnant by the time we left that I felt the stirrings of symptoms making me nauseous on the ride home. All I ended up with that month was a can of ginger ale from a rest stop and no pink line to speak of. We were undeterred and kept at it, sure it would happen. Nothing we had ever wanted had been that far out of reach.

As the months passed, we doubled down and became slaves to my menstrual cycle. Our lovemaking lost spontaneity and felt more like preparing for an exam. We did our homework and practiced the most up-to-date, surefire methods to ensure a pregnancy. Still, each month like clockwork, I reached for a tampon and soon enough a tissue as well. There was no more lounging around naked reading the New York Times in bed after making love on a Sunday morning…we were all business. The doctors we visited told us the usual cliches:

"You are young."

"Be patient, it will happen."

"Just relax."

But I was shattered, embarrassed. For the first time in my life something was out of reach and there was no adult in the room to come in and save us. Howie and I couldn't comfort each other no matter how hard we tried. I alternated between crying into his shoulder while holding on tight and pushing everyone, including him, as far away as possible.

Everyone annoyed me with their well-meaning, but hollow advice offered while toting a toddler on their hip. The most infuriating being, *just relax, it'll happen.* You try relaxing while rushing from intimacy to acrobatics to hiking your legs over your head for twenty minutes in the hopes of helping the swimmers find their way upstream for a match made in Stacy. Luckily, I had enough grace to keep my thoughts to myself.

I went from feeling like we had the world at our fingertips to wondering if we had a future at all. Starting a family and having a baby was what we always wanted, something we discussed, and part of my overall plan. But for the first time in my life, I couldn't check the box.

Once we passed the one-year mark, we began fertility treatment. We were living in subsidized housing in New York City while Howie completed two years of Oncology research. The doctor offered me a place in his support group. I never even considered it. I couldn't imagine anything worse than sitting with a group of people as sad and angry as I was. I had grown to hate the pity I saw in others' eyes and refused to allow their reflection to become reality.

Even at my worst, I fought to feel better, but it took all my strength to deal with my own situation. I couldn't fathom how I could take on others, and I knew I couldn't ever listen without doing just that. I never even spoke to other patients in the waiting room, even though many women were chatting and even exchanging phone numbers. I sat at attention, focused on picking my cuticles and whatever sentence I was reading over and over again until I was called into the office.

The doctors were hopeful and that was contagious at times. But for the most part, my mood, social life, and even my choice in clothing was dictated by a series of 28-day cycles marked by drugs, shots, procedures, tests, waiting periods…repeat. For those weeks when I was most fertile until the end of month, I was hopeful, trying to protect myself with as watered down a version of excitement as I could muster. On those last few days before my period, I shook so badly I carried a cup of coffee in one hand and a diet coke in the other around the office hoping to anchor my hands. Between treatment and nerves, I felt like a visitor in my own body. I wondered if anyone noticed my perpetually bloated stomach, the premature hot flashes, or could hear the blood pounding in my ears so loud that I took to sitting up front at meetings. I welcomed the advent of interoffice email so I could hide behind communications typed by my shaking hands.

The routine of work became comforting in its predictability. It was weekends and social plans with a growing number of friends becoming families that were the most painful. Outside of doctor appointments, our calendar was marked by self-inflicted attendance at social events of our age group: namings, brises, and first birthday parties. I was determined not to be absent from milestones for people who would be part of our life long after this was all over. I believed missing these events marginalized us even more than we already were, yet each one was a reminder all we brought to the party was a gift-wrapped present in otherwise empty arms.

There were times I simply couldn't perform. One Chanukah, Howie insisted I go to his Aunt Sheila's, where his cousin Tracy would be, pregnant with her first child. I gave in but was so angry he forced me that I boiled over when we got there. I barely spoke to Tracy and ignored her baby bump as best I could. I walked off periodically to cry in the bathroom and couldn't enjoy Aunt Sheila's famous latkes for the lump lodged in my throat. No one spoke of it until I apologized to Tracy years later, but the elephant in the room was there.

Howie and I were luckier than many in that we turned toward rather than away from each other. It wasn't easy. But we were dedicated to our relationship and worked at it. We knew it was the only way we would survive. Barely five years since we said I do and the latter part of *for better or worse* seemed relentlessly on repeat like a record needle unable to skip past a lone thread. It was a lot to handle, and we knew we needed help. We began seeing a therapist. We lived on the East Side, so heading all the way to the West Side for therapy seemed like another world to us. It was the perfect escape.

We held hands as we got out of the cab for that first appointment. I checked the address I had scribbled on the inside of a gum wrapper. There it was, West 77th Street, overlooking Central Park. I remember noting how much longer the blocks were than on the East Side. I liked the anonymity the wider sidewalks and taller buildings offered. My private life felt so exposed these days as family and friends had either caught on and asked enough questions to confirm their suspicions, or were part of a select few we invited into our world. It was difficult letting people in. It came with a reporting responsibility that I was rarely up for. As months passed, the circle of those in the know widened, some out of choice and some out of necessity. I recently had to tell my boss at work, as daytime doctor's appointments continued to pile up. Thankfully, the only emotion I sensed from her was a practiced tolerance for any requested time off, much easier to handle than the pity I saw in so many others. As we entered the therapist's office, I left any remnants of work and home at the door and focused on why we came.

Huddled together in the middle of her couch, we talked openly about our pain, our fears, and even dabbled in cracks in our relationship. Most of them surface-damage relating to treatment, but some ran deeper and could have easily shaken our foundation in years to come. Slowly, we found strength as a couple and solidified our vows to take care of each other. What stands out most from our time in her small, street-level office was the comfort of being there and the tools we learned to take back to our daily lives.

Therapy gave me insight, but it also gave me back some control. I felt healthier. Of course, the crashes happened each month, and I was angry at the world on some level most of the time. But over the next year, I learned how to cope. I chose who to let in and found the voice to tell others it was none of their business. I found strength to celebrate pregnancies and births selectively. I knew our close friend's daughter would only have one first birthday and I wanted to be there, so I was. But I also knew I couldn't go to a baby naming of an acquaintance the day after getting bad news, so I didn't.

Our therapist suggested we plan things that make us happy in preparation for days we receive news during our cycles. We loved to eat and were living in a foodie's paradise, so we took that one and ran with it. Date nights were born. I planned dinners to cook at home and timed them for nights we would get test results. If it was good news, we were ready to celebrate. If it was bad news, I had the perfect distraction and dove into cooking a meal we could both enjoy.

Howie planned romantic dinners at places we couldn't afford but went anyway. One in particular stands out. He told me to meet him on the steps of the Plaza, ready for a night out. I showed up from work to find him in a tuxedo with a dozen roses, ready to sweep me off my feet. We had drinks in the bar before heading to Aureole, one of the best restaurants in New York in the early '90s. He was so excited, but I couldn't stop laughing. In my role at Revlon, I chose restaurants for corporate events and frequently sampled menus at 5-star restaurants. That very afternoon I had been to Aureole! Not wanting to ruin his plans, I managed to shove five more stars into my stomach that evening.

Our trips to the therapist became date nights of their own. We left each session lost in our own thoughts, not quite ready to head East again. Instead, we'd wander the streets of the West Side hand in hand, my legs needing two steps for each one of his, remaining in sync block after block, night after night. Eventually we'd stop for dinner, sharing a comfortable silence usually reserved for couples married much longer. When we finally headed home, we were just better enough to face the next day.

While our date nights and dinners didn't solve our problems, they were a respite and a reset during one of our weakest times, setting a tone for the rest of our marriage.

After two full years, we were almost ready to wave the white flag on our fertility and change directions. Howie was there before me. It was the tiniest of creatures who gave me the final push.

Late one afternoon, Gail, also living in New York City, dropped off her six-month-old son so she could go to a doctor's appointment. As she set Brian on our bed and gave me the short list of instructions, I hoped I gave off an air of confidence I wasn't feeling. There were so many other friends she could have left him with—friends who had kids of their own—yet she chose me. I tried to act like it was no big deal, but my best friend, my first phone call after Howie, knew better.

I could hear the front door close followed by the sounds of the elevator doors opening. I knelt down so I was eye level with Brian, who was intent on mastering a baby pushup. I admired him. His belief anything could be achieved with sheer determination, still so pure and unmarred. Each time he found himself face first in the mattress, he barely missed a beat before his little arms started trying again.

Taking a deep breath, I reached over and picked him up. I kissed the top of his head as he settled into my arms. I could still smell the baby shampoo from last night's bath.

I started reading him one of the hard cover books Gail left behind. When he began falling forward into the book, I realized my storytelling was lulling him to sleep and I relaxed along with him.

We stayed that way for a long time, the late afternoon shadows creeping across the floor as I held tightly and watched him sleep. When I could barely see him in my arms anymore, I laid him gently on the bed and wiped my wet cheeks.

It took this tiny baby to give me a clarity I had been searching for. Caught in a seemingly endless cycle of fertility treatments, I had lost sight of what I really wanted. At that moment, watching Brian sleep, I realized I wanted to be a mom way more than I cared about getting pregnant.

A short six months later, we adopted our baby girl Molly, and I was thrilled to put this turmoil behind us.

―― CHAPTER THREE ――

And Baby Makes Three

Accepting I may never feel a baby kicking in my stomach or see a version of my eyes looking up at me begging for more chicken fingers seemed like a no brainer now that we were here.

For over two years, I watched from the sidelines as friend after friend announced their good news, sharing conception stories as if family planning was a given. I hung on, nodding along as if I were interested and not embarrassed by the burn of jealousy I felt at every word. I hoped the smiles and hugs I gave were enough to bridge the gap.

It was finally my turn. I knew all the stories of adoptions gone bad, birth parents changing their mind at the last minute.

"Don't get excited," my mom warned, "I don't want you to be let down if it doesn't work out."

That seemed impossible, and a waste of what could be an exciting and memorable time in our life. Yes, I had a flat belly, no OBGYN appointments on the calendar, and my breasts were the same 34B they had been since I bought my first bra, but we were having a baby! Why shouldn't I yell it from the rooftops? There was no real way to protect myself if things didn't work out. If our fertility treatment had taught me anything, I had learned that the depths I had to crawl out of each month when I got my period were no shallower if I didn't let myself dream.

I told everyone we met that we were expecting. Before long, it felt real, and I became comfortable, almost eager to answer the inquiring eyes as they searched for a baby bump.

"We're adopting. She's due in March." My smile answered any other questions.

Molly was born in March 1996 in Colville, Washington, a small town 30 miles south of the Canadian border. It was a beautiful morning. One of those days that you believe, no, one of those days you *know*, dreams are possible.

My childhood allowed me to dream big and believe in fairytales until an unexpected plot twist caught me off guard. But I was confident it was all over now. Surely the infertility had given me the battle scars of experience and earned me rightful passage to adulthood. In fact, if I was grading myself, I would give myself an A+, more reminiscent of high school grades than when life threw me a curve ball during the first semester of freshman year.

The grades were posted by student ID. I stopped by with Howie. We studied together. He was pre-med and very serious. While he spent our time studying with his head buried in his book, I spent my time watching him and doodling our initials together in hearts all over my notebook.

When it was our turn to find our grades, he went first. I watched him use his pointer finger to find his student ID and trace a line across to his grade.

"I got an A!" he announced proudly.

I confidently stepped forward, quickly locating my ID with my own pointer and dragged it across, my finger slowing down as my eyes arrived first. I blinked my eyes and stared. I couldn't believe it. A C? I had never gotten a C. How did this happen? I checked so many times I almost ripped a hole in the paper, but no matter how many times I traced that line the grade was the same.

I knew the justification—*at a school where everyone graduated at the top of their high schools, the natural bell curve will put some of us in the middle. C students.* I understood that. But something my father always said kept running through my head.

"If you can look me in the eye and tell me you did your best then that's all I can ever ask."

I was glad he wasn't here.

That afternoon I sat down alone in the library and made my first of many study lists. I planned out every day between then and the next set of tests, listing each subject, getting as specific as possible.

Tuesday 9–11 — Psych 101, outline chapters 1–3, summarize, make index cards.

I relaxed a little more with each task I assigned.

Making lists became a coping skill from that day forward. Breaking things down and putting them in writing helped make even the most daunting days seem manageable. To this day they help me plan, help me clear my head, and even on the most out of control days a single check mark can make me feel as if I accomplished something.

Molly's arrival meant many things to me. I was becoming a mother. *Check!* We were becoming a family. *Check!* We could put our fertility treatment, and all the painful memories, behind us. *Check! Check!* All we had left was to get through the final leg of the adoption.

We had arrived two weeks before the due date at the encouragement of Dan and Jill, Molly's birth parents. This was not their first child, and they insisted she would be early. For anyone who's been on the receiving end of an adoption, you don't question the person who is carrying your future, you react. We tied up things in New York City, both of us taking leave from our jobs, and boarded a plane to fly across the country. We had been to Colville twice before. The first time to meet Dan and Jill and sign the pre-adoption paperwork, and the second to go to a doctor's appointment and meet the team who would deliver our daughter.

Colville was beautiful by many standards. A tiny logging town where everyone seemed to know each other, and I came to understand our plans to adopt one of their own was big news. From the moment we arrived, many followed our progress over coffee in the downtown diner. We were staying in Maple on 6th, Colville's only bed and breakfast. Owners, Lois and Lee, greeted us as hosts and transformed quickly into surrogate parents inviting us to join them in the kitchen for not just breakfast, but lunch and dinner as well. By the time Molly arrived, Lois had added a bassinet, stuffed animals, and a freshly knitted comforter to our white lace, antique-filled room. The dreamlike setting was a stark contrast to the trailer park and chaotic life of Dan and Jill where we spent much of the time waiting for Molly to be born.

Adoption laws vary by state, and we were working with attorneys in both New York and in Washington. The one in Washington was a kind, laid back man, who was handling all the money between us and the birth parents. We were not allowed to give them money directly, as that could be considered buying a baby. Everything flowed through the attorney. That doesn't mean we weren't taken advantage of—we unquestioningly paid anything the attorney approved for the entirety of the pregnancy, including extras such as bailing Dan out of jail for a misdemeanor and helping them find a new trailer to move to.

From the beginning, they seemed more attached to us than to the baby that brought us together.

"You guys will make the best parents. You are exactly the kind of people we want for this one. She's going to be special. I can feel it. She kicked today. I can't wait for you to come out here so you can feel it yourself. When are you coming? Not till then? Why not? We miss you guys!"

We were afraid to let them down, so night after night in the months leading up to the adoption, we listened to their stories from the 800 number we set up in our apartment. For hours at a time we were trapped on the phone while they rambled on, barely taking a breath, much like a child recounts a day at school.

"We woke up and ate lunch. I made macaroni and cheese. Dan spent the day playing videos with his friend who lives in the next trailer. The dog wouldn't leave him alone. Probably because he had to go out. He damn near beat the dog. I have to keep *(the dog)* away from him when he's playing, or he'll kill the poor thing!"

While we were very close in age, it became clear we were the only adults in the room. They were both immature to a fault with no real sense of responsibility. Not to themselves and barely to the baby they were still in charge of. They changed their phone number instead of paying the bill, did much the same for cable, changed their names to sign up for new credit cards, and moved homes before they could be tracked down. They didn't work at all while we knew them but talked about jobs they had where they were wronged, overqualified, underappreciated, or injured and collected disability checks. Since we were supporting them during this time, it was hard to know if they ever worked or lived off disability checks and sold the occasional household items to the local pawn shop as needed. They smoked cigarettes and claimed that was the extent of their substance use.

They held all the cards, and they knew it. They fed our egos telling us what we wanted to hear mixed with veiled threats emphasizing their power. We waited anxiously for their calls, convinced they'd change their minds or disappear at any sign of trouble.

While we couldn't be there the whole time we compensated with creative cross-country touches as much as we could. At Christmas I filled two big bags with gifts for each of them. Colorfully packaged games and gifts that I still remember to this day. Jenga, drawing paper, colored markers, pens, writing paper, and a small keyboard for her. Video games for him.

I tried not to think about how difficult it was to be with them, or how little control I had, or the unfairness of the whole situation, because, at the end of the day, we were going to be parents. The irony was not lost on me that the very people I may have hurried past on the streets a few months earlier had become the ones who we were counting on to make our deepest dreams come true.

As the birth date grew closer, I needed to address what would happen *after*.

"Are we going to get to talk to you and Howard after Molly is born?" Jill asked me one afternoon.

Keeping the tremble out of my voice, I tried to be both gentle and firm reminding her of our earlier conversations.

"We agreed it is best for Molly if we do not speak and instead send you yearly updates, tell her about you, and leave it up to her when she is older."

I could hear the little girl whine replaced by someone who knows her power and it terrified me. Revealing what she was capable of shrouded in the wisdom of her experience in this area. She showed us what she could do if we misstepped.

"Well, I'm really going to miss you. In fact, I'm getting very upset thinking about giving up Molly at all. Now I'm not changing my mind; I'm just telling you what I've been feeling. It's normal to feel this way at the end of a pregnancy. I always have second thoughts. I never go back on my word though. I haven't yet. But I always thought I'd keep this one. But I know you and Howard will be such great parents—that's what's keeping me from changing my mind this time. You and Howard and how great you are to us."

I couldn't wait for it to be over.

Molly was born on March 7, one week after she was due. Howie and I were both in the delivery room. In fact, as a third-year surgical resident, the doctor allowed Howie to deliver our daughter! The whole town seemed to pitch in to make our transition to parenthood as easy and exciting as possible. We were the only family on the maternity ward that day and the hospital allowed us to stay in a room overnight. The local pizza parlor sent in dinner, and a bouquet of balloons arrived with Lois and Lee.

Jill enjoyed her private room and the attention she got from her own nurses, but didn't ask to see Molly that night or the next morning before she went home. Dan came to our room in the hospital but only to give us a report on Jill before heading back to their room with some slices of pizza.

I first held Molly in the delivery room, but it wasn't until I was in our own room holding her on my chest, skin to skin, with Dan and Jill on the other side of the hospital, that I felt the connection I had been dreaming of for years. She was ours…almost.

Before Molly's adoption could be finalized and we could go home with her, we had to:

1. *Wait the longest forty-eight hours of my life, during which either Dan or Jill could change their minds.*

2. *Be observed and approved as fit by a state-appointed social worker.*
3. *Go before a judge.*

After a sleepless night of taking turns holding and staring at Molly, we left the hospital and went back to Maple on 6th to hold our breath for another thirty-two hours (*but who was counting?*).

Our parents arranged with Lois to have more balloons, flowers, and a pile of baby gifts waiting for us. Lois, excited herself to have a baby in the house, offered to hold Molly while we slept. It was a kind gesture, but we were more than ready to dive into child rearing and welcomed the distraction from watching the hands on the clock count down.

The social worker was scheduled to come over the next morning. The irony of Howie and I being judged on our parenting skills, when our daughter would've been left in a dirty trailer where violence was the norm and drugs a possibility, was not lost on us. I reminded myself that it didn't matter anymore. Molly was ours.

Before the social worker came to meet with us, we thought we'd give Molly her first bath. It was also our first time giving a bath to a newborn, so I prepared as any good student would; I brought directions!

We cleared the shelf in the bathroom set up more for a good long soak than the bathing of a newborn. We put the plastic tub next to the sink and filled it with warm water. We put the directions in front of us. We decided Howie would read and I would do the bathing.

"Check the water," he began.

We checked the water. It was just warm enough.

We continued to follow the directions instructing us to sponge off each body part individually so she wouldn't get too cold. Once clean, we toweled her dry and returned her, limb by limb, to new clothes. We were so caught up we barely noticed when the transformation was complete.

Unfortunately, we forgot something. We had to clip her nails.

"I got this," Howie said.

I let my husband, new father, and *surgeon*, clip my newborn daughter's nails as I began to clean up. What could possibly go wrong?

"Oh shit!" I heard from behind me.

Molly's cries followed immediately.

I turned around to see Howie frantically wiping up blood that seemed to be coming from Molly's thumb and quickly covering her clean pajamas. To any other parents, this probably wouldn't be such a big deal, but to two parents facing evaluation by a social worker on their parenting ability, it felt nothing less than tragic.

Before long, Molly's finger stopped bleeding. I took out a new outfit, and together we cleaned up and dressed her. She calmed down, and it was at this moment, with the three of us standing in the bathroom in the bed and breakfast, across the country from our family, awaiting a social worker's approval, that we began to laugh. With that laughter my insecurities about motherhood that my infertility had bred began to subside. I had a long way to go, but I started to realize-

This is my family,

I am a mother, and this is our journey now.

With a passing grade from the social worker and barely an hour left until the waiting period was over, we began to relax. To talk about flights home and plans when we got there. It was right around this time that Dan paid us a visit.

We heard the doorbell ring and Lee opening the door. Muffled voices, but we knew. We left Molly sleeping just in time to see Dan climbing the white carpeted steps, tracking mud from his work boots without giving it a thought. Those footprints seemed to highlight the contrast between what could have been for Molly and what we hoped to give her from this day forward.

When Dan saw us, he broke out in a big smile like he found his long-lost friends.

"Hey, you guys! I missed you. Jill is home resting and wanted me to come over and find out when we're going to see you. We're hungry and wondered what you're eating for dinner. We were worried you'd leave without saying goodbye."

No mention of changing their mind. No mention of Molly at all.

We told him how busy we'd been taking care of Molly, but quickly turned the attention back to them, asking how Jill was feeling. I realized they were not changing their mind and as the relief washed over me, I let it out in a torrent of gratitude for what they had given us.

"She's everything we've been dreaming of. She's perfect. We couldn't be happier. And it's all because of you and Jill! We are glad she's feeling okay. Please give her a hug for us."

He seemed a little let down we didn't head back to the trailer right then, or at least buy him dinner, but he gave us quick hugs and left.

That visit made us both uncomfortable. It was clear Dan and Jill were more interested in us then the child they gave birth to. And we knew that interest was, for the most part, financial. While they couldn't change their minds after the waiting period, we didn't trust them. Once the adoption was complete, our financial support was ending. We didn't know everything they were capable of but had seen enough to be concerned they'd do whatever they could to stay as comfortable as we'd made them for the past five months.

We decided it was best for us and for Molly to cut ties with Dan and Jill as quickly as possible. We had a baby to worry about now. A short two days later, we left Dan and Jill a letter thanking them but stopping short of promising to stay in touch. We disconnected our 800 number when we got home and never sent any updates. It was a hard decision, but one I would make again, especially after calling the attorney a few months later. We learned Dan and Jill went to his office just once after we left. They said they tried to call us, and when they couldn't reach us, they decided to go into the office to find out if we left them any money. That was it.

We planned to and did tell Molly she was adopted from the moment she could understand. "My belly was broken, so your birth mother grew you for me. And then the doctors really fixed it so I could grow two babies!" was the story she learned and repeated to anyone who would listen.

After a judge in Spokane finalized our adoption, our family boarded a flight together to New York to go home.

When the flight attendant commented on how good I looked considering I gave birth only five days earlier, I realized there were some perks of adopting I hadn't even thought of!

We were welcomed into our old/new life by our extended family, complete with signs and more balloons, and flowers at the gate. I quickly lost sight of Molly as she was passed from grandparents to great grandparents, aunts and uncles. It didn't end there. Our small apartment was filled with friends, still more balloons, and baby gifts from everyone ranging from close friends to work acquaintances. I was finally able to let in the love and support that I'd read as pity so many times over the past two years. In many ways it was like I re-entered my life, and I was glad to be back, joined by our little girl who made me a mommy.

Molly saved us. She made it possible to move forward. She brought lightness back into our lives. She had the cutest chubby baby legs and blonde hair, a giggle that instantly made you laugh along, and a smile that could light the whole sky. But I still felt a step behind the other moms who planned their pregnancies and made it all look so easy. I knew there was no Scarlet A for adoption on me, but I couldn't shake the feeling I stood out.

I thought meeting other moms with babies the same age would help. Molly was just six weeks old, and the class was for newborns to three months. When I tried to sign up for the Mommy and Me Class at the local hospital, I was told that classes were only for mothers who gave birth at that hospital. The unfairness enraged me enough to overcome any feelings of inadequacy. I kept at it, explaining over and over to faceless admins on the other end of the phone.

"But I didn't give birth at all. I adopted our daughter in Washington State."

Finally, someone begrudgingly relented. Much like the adopting, it didn't matter how we joined the class—we were in!

I was proud I made it happen. Still, while lying awake in bed in the middle of the night, I counted my insecurities like sheep.

1. *I didn't give birth at the hospital hosting the class.*
2. *I didn't give birth at all!*
3. *Did I deserve to be a mother?*
4. *Were there things they knew that I didn't?*
5. *Should I tell anyone Molly was adopted?*
6. *What would they think?*
7. *Would they know just by looking at us?*
8. *Would my name have an asterisk on the list at the class?*

The Mommy and Me class began at 11:00 a.m. I began preparing the night before and now, with barely an hour to go, I was finally ready. My *"don't leave the apartment without"* list lay next to my keys in the foyer. My new diaper bag sat stuffed and ready under the blue Peg Perego at the door, patiently waiting for me to load Molly into it, ride the elevator downstairs, and walk the short six blocks to Cornell Medical Center.

Molly was still sleeping from her morning nap, so I transferred her to the carriage and left the apartment. My confidence built with every step, and I looked up into the late April sun, breathing in the scent of spring and smiling at nothing in particular.

I found my way to the class, noting I was in the same building where I had gotten fertility injections for almost two years. Stopping short of talking to myself in the elevator, I nodded away any doubts, reminding myself I belonged there before stepping into a room filled with identical carriages, their passengers lying comfortably with their mothers in a circle on the floor. I made my way over to an empty spot and busied myself by unbuckling a still sleeping Molly and lifting her out. As I sat down, the conversation flowed easily.

"How old is she?"

"She's so cute, how is she sleeping?"

"Has she eaten today?"

My heart dropped. *Eaten. Uh oh.*

With a sense of dread I got up, holding Molly in one arm, and silently praying she stayed asleep. I reached into my diaper bag and felt around, already knowing I wouldn't find it. My heart sank. I had forgotten a bottle.

I resisted the overwhelming urge to turn and run. If Molly woke and was hungry, which she most definitely would be, I had no way to soothe her. I couldn't breastfeed like many of these moms. *What kind of mother forgets her child's bottle?*

I could barely hear the moderator over my heart pounding, but as class wore on and Molly slept, I relaxed and even participated by telling the group my unique birthing story. Their questions were born of pure interest and made me feel less like a side show with each passing moment. But it wasn't until weeks later, when these strangers became friends, that I was able to laugh about forgetting a bottle to my first Mommy and Me Class.

Being Molly's mom saved me from myself. The need to check all the boxes and do everything perfectly. Slowly I learned that is not real life. Real life is forgetting bottles. Check! Navigating with grace, or at least trying to, when things don't go as planned Check! Laughing at yourself. Check! Check!

I learned a lot those first few years of motherhood from Molly, and still more three years and a twin pregnancy later, from Leo and Emily. When Howie completed his surgical training, we moved to Pennsylvania where he began his practice as a colon and rectal surgeon. With my family complete I was ready to settle down and make memories in what was to be a storybook life.

—— CHAPTER FOUR ——

Finding Mrs. Fix-It

Step…Pause…Step…Pause. I smiled, picturing her stopping on each step with two feet to regain her four-year-old balance. Her blonde hair swinging and her chubby hands grazing the walls as she took the three-floor journey. She was still getting used to the steps in our new home, and I was glad she was taking her time.

We had just moved into the three-story stone colonial on the Main Line of Philadelphia. From the moment I stepped into the house I knew this was it. Sitting sideways on a tree-lined street, only one block away from the train station, the neighborhood had as much charm as the house itself. Filled with children navigating the well-worn, uneven sidewalks, trailed behind by mothers with single and double strollers, I knew I would find much more than a house here. It had all the possibilities of becoming the home I so yearned for. After moving six times during Howie's medical training, I was more than ready to set down roots.

Step…Pause…Step…Pause.

Four years of medical school, seven years of residency, and

a year of fellowship training. For twelve years Howie's training had dictated where we lived and how often we moved. He finally began his first full-time job just a few weeks ago. Between long deferred loan repayments and a newly acquired mortgage, we still barely made it each month. Luckily our new home didn't need much immediate attention. Some childproofing, a fresh coat of paint, and a new carpet to soften the 1923 original hardwood, and we were good to go.

We settled into our new life immediately. I was invited to a neighborhood playgroup where, among others, I met the other five sets of twins on the block! When Molly began kindergarten in September, I joined the crowd at the bus stop every morning. The bus stop was an event in itself. Like a scene out of Mayberry, our doors all opened within minutes of each other and kids flowed toward the designated corner, some with backpacks ready for the bus ride to elementary school, others still toting bottles, and still others hiked on the hip of their moms. We talked, laughed, and commiserated long after the bus pulled away, sometimes so caught up in relaying last night's bedtime catastrophe that we forgot to wave goodbye to our elementary schooler. It wasn't long before we became each other's emergency contacts and spent many holidays together. We hosted a New Year's Eve family potluck party each year. Before everyone came, we turned the clocks ahead two and a half hours. At precisely 9:30 p.m. Howie appeared at the top of the steps in a tuxedo and dropped a homemade ball. We cheered, we threw confetti, and we banged pots and pans. And we were all home and in our beds shortly after 10:00 p.m.! We had a neighborhood dinner club for adults only, but most of our social life included our kids.

On Friday afternoons we met in one backyard filled with snacks for the kids and drinks for us. As the afternoon waned, we took turns counting heads, sometimes organizing a game but mostly reveling in how lucky we were to have each other. Slowly we discussed dinner, ordering pizza or turning on a barbecue, and the husbands eventually showed up some with briefcases in hand straight from the train station down the block, others in comfortable clothes having stopped at home before following the sounds of laughter.

Step…Pause…Step…Pause.

I listened to Molly continue her journey while keeping a hand on each of the slippery two-year-olds in the bathtub.

Molly was supposed to stay downstairs with Terry, our new babysitter. Earlier, we gave all three kids dinner together, and after that I followed Leo and Emily as they climbed up the steps in their diapers, their clothes left in their highchairs full of jarred carrots and sweet potatoes.

The twins were busy giggling and talking to each other in their own language as they did whenever they were in the bathtub. Their laughter was contagious, Leo's beginning in his belly and Emmy's much more delicate like a series of hiccups. However, I found it difficult to focus and enjoy this moment of just being with them. I couldn't let go of a gnawing discomfort deep in my belly that I was slowly becoming familiar with whenever I left Molly with someone else. It wasn't anything I could put my finger on yet, and I was hesitant to sound too many alarms. It's hard to know when it's your firstborn how atypical behaviors such as cutting the hair off a friend's Barbie at a playdate, jumping up and down in a sink in the bathroom at a pizza parlor *(until it came out of the wall)*, or telling the babysitter they have permission to fingerpaint on the walls of the playroom, really are for a four-year-old girl. All I know is that lately, every time we were apart, I got a phone call.

As I struggled with this unnerving feeling, I looked at the twins so full of life and thought back to the day I found out I was pregnant. While I had made peace with the possibility of never giving birth myself, our doctors advised we try again. We were still young, and our infertility was deemed *unexplained*, doctor speak for *we really don't know what is wrong*. We had been through it all before and knew what to expect. And if it didn't work? We'd adopt again. We were more than okay with that!

Now that we were several cycles in, the hormone highs and lows were starting to wear on me, and I wondered how many more I could handle before I'd give the green light on adoption again. While I was okay with either path to parenthood, I hadn't fully given up on becoming pregnant and giving birth. It wasn't something I said out loud, but late at night after Molly was asleep in her crib, I fantasized about just reaching for Howie and making a baby. For many, getting pregnant was just that simple. For us, it included teams of doctors, injections, and procedures. The adoption was complicated as well. I'd love to be done with it all and still have the family I wanted.

I was holed up in my office, yet fully exposed in my glass cubicle in the center of my department. As vice president of corporate communications, I had a 360 view of the staff working to support the insurance company we worked for. On this day, among the many problems thrown at me every day, loomed the one I was yet unable to solve. I knew I would hear any minute and was trying to bury myself in my work. But no matter how absorbed I thought I became, only minutes passed each time I glanced at the clock. It was torture. I choked down a quick lunch in the cafeteria only to rush back to my office and wait some more.

I knew the results of my blood test were waiting for a nurse, who was most likely working through a pile of call backs, to pick up the phone and deliver life changing news.

There it was. The red light was blinking, indicating a call for my extension. I looked at it for a few seconds, suddenly frozen. There was so much at stake, and I wanted to stay in this place of possibility for a little longer. When I knew I risked them hanging up or getting lost in our corporate message system, I answered.

"Corporate Communications, Stacy speaking."

"Is this my beautiful wife?"

My heart sank. It was just Howie. He never seemed as paralyzed as me during these waiting periods. He sounded way too cheerful for me right now, and I couldn't wait to get off the phone.

"I haven't heard anything yet. Can I call you back?"

"Sure. I just wanted to see if you had time for lunch."

Why was he asking me this? I realized he must know something. As a surgical resident, he was able to call the lab and get results. I'd been down this road before. He must want to come and soften the blow.

"I already ate. Just tell me if you know something. I can't take it anymore."

"Well, did you feel like you were eating for two?"

My world stopped. I let his words sink in.

"What are you talking about?" I asked shakily, afraid of the answer.

"I called the lab, and your numbers show positive—you, I mean we, are pregnant!"

I scooted my chair to the corner of my office between two file cabinets, the most private space available, and covered my face with both hands, heaving cries of relief while I asked Howie to repeat it over and over.

"Are you sure?" I think I may have even squealed.

"Yes, sweetie, I'm sure. We are pregnant."

"Can I take another test to be sure?"

"You can take as many tests as you want!"

"What do we do now?"

"Nothing, finish your day, and we will celebrate tonight."

That seemed impossible. I knew I couldn't tell anyone at work yet, and the glass cubicle made it impossible for a private phone call. How was I to walk around with this news bubbling inside of me threatening to pop like the *(non-alcoholic)* champagne bottle I couldn't wait to open tonight? I convinced Howie to drive the fifteen minutes to my office so I could climb into his car for a few minutes, where I exploded in a torrent of tears and excitement. I didn't know what lay ahead, but I knew enough to absorb these moments of joy while I had them.

Soon we found out we were pregnant with not just one baby, but two. And nine months later they were born.

Family of five. *Check!*

Step…Pause…Step…Pause…

Molly reached the third-floor landing and was just outside the bathroom door.

Suddenly, the twins pointed and giggled at the door to the bathroom. In my high-pitched mommy voice I began, "Is that your big sister, Molly?" But as I turned around, keeping a hand on each twin in the tub, I stopped speaking and opened my eyes so wide my contacts almost fell out. Standing before me was Molly but not as I had left her in the kitchen. No…this Molly was completely naked and completely painted purple. I'm not just talking about light strokes all over. When I say completely purple, I mean every crevasse imaginable had been touched by a paint brush, as well as hands and bottom of feet. The bottom of her feet!

I quickly lifted the twins out of the tub, holding them like footballs in each arm and ran to the top of the steps. It was worse than I had imagined…purple footsteps covered the newly laid carpet marking the path Molly had just made, and four-year-old handprints marked her journey on our newly painted walls. I won't pretend I kept my cool. Any sweetness in my voice turned sour as I turned on her.

"Why did you do this?"

Unaffected by my yelling, she came over and hugged me purple, answering, "I'm a present, Mommy. I'm a purple dinosaur present for you!"

I knew it was cute, and I knew it was funny. But I didn't laugh until much, much later. I put them all in the bath together and cleaned Molly up too. Luckily it took just a little extra scrubbing and she was clean.

After the bath, I said goodbye to Terry, who had been cleaning the kitchen and seemed shocked at what had transpired, forever! I got to work and before long the purple dinosaur prints were a distant memory. That night I laid down with Molly as she fell asleep. She looked so peaceful. It was hard to believe the trail of chaos this little girl could leave in her wake. For a child who moved a mile a minute for the rest of the day, once she became focused on a story, she put her thumb in her mouth, drew her blanket in close with her other hand, and snuggled onto my shoulder, releasing any four- year-old tension with one deep breath.

As I read, she periodically removed her thumb with a pop and pointed to a picture asking a question about a character or the story itself. She put her hand on the page, trying to physically connect with the characters and leaving a wet mark before returning the thumb to its place of comfort and letting me continue.

Bright as anything, she stopped me with her blanket in hand and turned the pages back, noting any inconsistencies in the storyline. Listening to her wonder how a wicked stepmother could possibly have ice in her veins when "everyone knows it's blood that runs through our veins" was both entertaining and mind boggling. I always took her questions seriously. After all, to quote a favorite family movie, *Stepbrothers*, "medicine is the family business." I wondered if these questions were the impulse of an innocent child or a creative procrastination technique. Either way, it was our ritual, and I willingly played my part. Every time.

Most remarkable was that just when I noticed her lengthened breaths and closed eyes and thought she had fallen asleep, she asked another question, barely understandable through the thumb still firmly in her mouth.

She fell asleep on my shoulder, and we sat there peacefully for what seemed like hours before I slid out from under her carefully, placing her head on her pillow. Her blanket was grasped as tightly as the thumb in her mouth. I stayed there for a few minutes trying to see her room through her eyes.

A twin trundle bed chosen with plans of sleepovers in mind, tucked in the corner and covered in a comforter of pastel pinks, yellows, and greens. Matching valences adorned both windows connected by the large, shabby chic dresser and matching hutch standing between them. Her night table matched as did the corner desk that sat unused but patiently knowing it would be busy in the years to come. A high-piled light beige rug made it cozy and soft and easy to jump from bed to floor without much risk. The walls were covered with pictures of princesses smiling at its inhabitant, and in case anyone was unsure, large painted wooden letters, spelling out MOLLY, hung over the bed.

I was very proud of how it came out. Each piece was chosen with love or made by hand given the very strict budget we were living under. It was the first room done in the house, and I hoped it gave her the peace she needed.

The day caught up with me and I decided to lie down again *just for a minute*. I closed my eyes only to be awakened by Molly stroking my cheek. I kept my eyes closed and held my breath, treasuring the closeness I felt with every feather light touch.

It wasn't long before her hand fell limply back onto the bed and her breathing signaled she was asleep again.

Our perfect family was not without its messes, but it felt like nothing a good bucket of soap, a lighthearted giggle, and a story time couldn't fix. And the fixer in me loved that.

A woman is like a teabag. You can't tell how strong she is until you put her in hot water.

-ELEANOR ROOSEVELT

PART TWO

Hanging On by a Thread

CHAPTER FIVE

A Fork in the Road

"Mrs. Ross? It's Susan Ellicot, the guidance counselor from Birch Street Middle School. I have Molly here."

As I pressed for details, I could hear the shuffling of Mrs. Ellicot moving to a place with more privacy. I waited. Then, in a strained whisper, "She is saying she doesn't want to live anymore and has thought about hurting herself."

My knees buckled and I went on autopilot. My mind went numb. I needed to get to Molly. With a speed and intent only known to parents desperate to protect their young, I tucked the phone between my ear and shoulder, picked up my keys, and was backing the car out of the driveway before Mrs. Ellicot finished describing the scene.

It was late fall of Molly's eighth grade year. She had been struggling since we moved from Philadelphia two years earlier, but it was difficult to know how aware she was of her own isolation. I hovered like a hawk ready to dive in at the first sign of trouble. But she didn't seem to notice the girls closing the circle as she approached, the weekends without the phone ringing, or the eyerolls as she passed almost anywhere in our small town.

Holding on to the wheel to stop my hands from shaking, I drove the short mile up the hill to her middle school in record time, grateful for the near empty streets and absent police force. The chatter in my head ping-ponged between self-blame and solutions. *How could I miss this? What caused this? What do we do now?* I didn't know she was in such turmoil, but I could certainly understand why.

I screeched to a stop in a double-lined zone and barely remembered to turn off the engine before jumping out of the car. Like I had been doing more and more frequently, I channeled my yoga training. My years of yoga taught me to be easy on myself during times like these. Understanding the interconnection between body, breath, and mind helped me find some peace from the growing chaos of my home life. Increasingly I found myself turning to my practice when life pushed my buttons, clearing my mind during savasana *(the ending pose of most classes)* allowing me to reset before facing the world again. Over the past two years I had embraced a yogic lifestyle, working to take my practice off my mat into every facet of my life. Taking pauses and breathing before impulsively reacting, searching for and finding silver linings where I couldn't before, and being easier on myself and those around me for daily missteps. But how could I prepare for what lay ahead of me right now? This was unchartered territory. I focused on what I could control: my breath. As if in a trance I watched my feet carry me into the school, one step at a time.

When I arrived at Mrs. Ellicot's office, a complacent Molly was sitting on a chair, her knees gathered into her too skinny arms and her head resting on her knees as if trying to make herself invisible. Usually, her large personality balanced out her small size but today was different. The sight of her rolled into a ball in the corner of the room began to crack my fragile composure. I tried to swallow past the lump in my throat.

Molly was on meds for ADHD for almost seven years. We knew the potential side effects of curbing her appetite and slowing her growth. We hoped to teach her to manage her symptoms while on the meds and eventually take her off them. We thought we were making progress, but right now I wasn't sure of anything. My little bundle of energy—I just wanted her to be the best version of herself.

Looking at her tucked in the corner, it was hard to believe she was ever considered big for her age. She was nine pounds, eleven ounces at birth. She didn't grow like a big baby and barely touched twenty pounds by her first birthday. Her larger birth size was probably due to her birth mother's gestational diabetes.

Her size made many things easier for us as first-time parents. She ate better, she slept longer—through the night at six weeks old. By the time she was born, most of our friends had children and she was the easiest baby by far.

Our parental honeymoon continued into toddlerhood. Molly sucked her thumb for comfort, and I ignored all advice to stop her. I didn't care. In fact, I came to expect the popping sound as she removed her thumb to speak, replacing it and removing it throughout conversations. She spoke early, stringing sentences together from her car seat in the minivan well before she was two.

On a crisp fall day as I was explaining why the leaves were falling and it was getting colder, *"Mommy, need sweater, cold out!"*

On a ride to meet my mother at a mall halfway between our homes for lunch, *"Mommy, shop till we drop!"* (I was teaching her well).

I watched her from the rear-view mirror. My little buddy. My smart, beautiful girl. Any worries I had about connecting with this child were long gone. I rambled on incessantly, narrating our life for her.

"Time for a bath. First let's take off these dirty clothes. Lift your arms. That's it. Now put your dress in the hamper. That's where we put the clothes that are dirty so we can clean them. We put you in the bathtub to clean you because little girls can't go into the washing machine. That would be silly. Now here we go, let's fill the bathtub…"

"We are going to school. Let me buckle you in. One buckle, now the other. Love you *(quick peck on the cheek)*. Now mommy is going to get in the driver's seat because I can't reach the wheel from back here!"

"Mommy is going to drop you at school where you'll get to play with your friends all day. And Mommy will go to work. But Mommy will be back because Mommy ALWAYS comes back…"

Before long, my speeches became conversations interspersed with giggles, kisses, and those chubby arms reaching for hugs. Even when the twins were born, we continued, just adding in comments about Leo and Emily to our discussions

Molly loved me, but she adored Howie. Daddy's little girl. She squealed when he came home, and as soon as her legs carried her, she ran to him. He'd lift her up and swing her around. She was tiny and light as a feather, and her laughter filled every corner of our household.

She either rode Howie's shoulders for much of every weekend, or she walked between us, reaching up to hold our hands. Howie and I would count to three and swing her high. Her pleas for more bringing smiles to our faces and everyone around us. We looked as happy as we were.

As she grew, Molly continued to stand out in a positive way. She was affectionate, empathetic, and early to most milestones. Even as she became difficult to slow down at night, I shrugged it off, describing her as "a light bulb that burns brightest before it goes out." I wonder sometimes if I described her that way hoping to find her behavior common and calm my suspicions. It didn't work.

Even as the first symptoms showed themselves, hyperactivity, impulse control issues, socially inappropriate behavior, I was able to manage them. I did get frustrated with her. Especially once the twins were there. But she melted me fast back then. Her antics were very often funny in hindsight. Once everyone was asleep, I had cleaned up and had a glass of wine in my hands. Yes, then very funny.

When the twins were born, we made a big deal about her being a big sister. She looked so cute in her *big sister present*—roller blades complete with knee pads, elbow pads, a helmet, and wrist guards. I may as well have wrapped her in bubble wrap! She never seemed jealous of them and instead wanted to be a part of every step. She sat with me topless in my room as I pumped breast milk, holding a cup she got from the kitchen up to her three-year-old chest, chatting non-stop about what was happening.

"Can I feed Leo and Emily too?"

"Why can't I give them milk from me?"

She sat for pictures, holding them, glowing from the praise of friends and family.

"What a great big sister!"

"You are so gentle with them!"

"They are going to look up to you."

"They love you already!"

One day we sat her on a chair and propped the three-month-old twins into sitting positions on either side of her for our first family picture with them *sitting up*. As we tried to take the picture, we cheered Molly on.

"Great job Molly!" I said with the voice of a very proud

mom. In her excitement she put her arms around each of them. We loved it.

"That's great!" Howie exclaimed, equally proud.

Then she took their heads and clunked them together in front of her still laughing. We weren't.

But once the twins stopped crying and we recovered, we looked at Molly, who was comforting both her siblings and apologizing.

"I didn't mean to clunk you, Leo. I love you, Emmy," she said in the sweetest voice.

We looked at the video we took along with the pictures and realized it was innocent, and we laughed.

That's the thing. Most, if not all her missteps when she was younger were innocent. Many of them were encouraged by family and friends. She liked the attention and couldn't seem to tell the difference between positive and negative attention. I was constantly trying to distinguish between what was normal for her age and any red flags. Her innocence and big blue eyes helped her get away with a lot and even get second chances.

I wondered if today's phone call could be another awkward attempt at attention. With high school looming, more and more was expected of her, yet no matter how many times I reviewed all the things that may have happened leading up to today, I fell short in understanding why she would threaten suicide.

We began to notice Molly was *different* when she started pre-school and had her first playdates. As the other girls were progressing to side-by-side play, Molly was still playing alone even when she had friends over. Her behavior was, at times, strange.

One mom called me mid-playdate explaining, "Molly is sitting in an empty bathtub playing alone."

Another one called upset: "Molly threw my daughter's Barbie doll out the window."

Still another sounded sorry. "I tried to get them to play together but she just played by herself." It wasn't long before Molly stopped being invited back to most houses and to most birthday parties.

Luckily, my network of *mom* friends with similar age kids made sure Molly's name wasn't crossed off every invitation list. For the others, I had all playdates at our house, where I watched and intervened before any doll had their hair cut or was thrown out a window.

In kindergarten the gap between Molly and the other girls widened. Her behavior was often unpredictable, and she had no sense of personal space. Even with social skills training classes, where they taught her to *respect the invisible hula hoop around everyone*, she barreled up to girls, grabbing them in an unwanted bear hug, missing all signals, even ignoring a clear *"Molly, stop."* Her handwriting was well below grade level, even though her reading and verbal skills were way above. The teacher kept saying she was a free spirit and insisted we had nothing to be concerned about.

But I knew better.

I was a straight A student until college. But even then, grades were important to me. As a young child I couldn't wait to show my parents my gold stars and still cringe at the few negative comments on my elementary school report cards. "Stacy's handwriting is illegible." "Still chatting away…" Howie was no different. It was hard to accept having a child who didn't seem to care about homework, and I didn't know if it was that or something else making it difficult for her to complete her work. I worried if she couldn't do those simple, short kindergarten assignments, how would she handle elementary school, high school, college?

All those worries seemed so minor after today's phone call. I listened to Mrs. Ellicot describe the events leading up to this moment. "Molly is missing homework assignments. And the ones that were handed in were late or incomplete. Her homework grade is a large part of her grade in several of her classes…"

As the stay-at-home parent, I saw overseeing the kids' homework each day as one of my responsibilities. Even as early as kindergarten, I had taken to trying different approaches with Molly.

I remember leaving Leo and Emily happily in front of the TV watching an episode of Caillou so I could work alone with Molly in her room. I ran through the day's plan like I was reviewing notes on index cards before an exam at college:

She's only a kid.
She's your daughter.
Remember who's in charge.
Go for it!

I took a deep breath, turned the knob, and peered around the door too tentatively. There she was center stage. A pink tutu and one of my bras put on over the clothes she wore to school that day. The dress-up trunk, a gift from my parents, flung open with the castaways from her search strewn across the floor. The winners, a veiled crown and matching wand, completed her outfit.

She was twirling around in a world all of her own, a soundtrack only she heard directing her from floor to bed and back, as graceful as a five-year-old can be. It would have been precious, but I only saw her intricate fantasy as a further obstacle.

I reminded myself I had planned for this and stepped inside. She barely noticed as she whirled past me. I stood firmly in front of her, catching her gaze until she put herself on pause.

"Hi, Mommy, I'm a fairy!"

I reached over and gently removed her crown, clearing the

wispy blonde bangs from her eyes. I squatted directly in front, keeping my hand firmly on her shoulder until I could see her blue eyes stop flitting around the room and meet my gaze.

"And you are a great fairy who can continue to dance as soon as your homework is done."

A flicker of understanding was replaced quickly by a light in her eyes. A new idea.

"Mommy, you can be a fairy too."

Did she even hear me? I wondered. I relaxed my jaw before it could fully clench.

"Maybe later. Right now, we must do your homework. The sooner we get started the sooner we will be done. "

I led her to her desk as she kept looking over her shoulder as if saying goodbye or trying to run away. We stopped at her backpack dropped on the floor next to the pajamas she had stepped out of that morning. Her whole day was laid out in front of me like a short story. I knelt down and unzipped the backpack, asking her to show me her homework.

After digging between notebooks, pencils, erasers, and balled up tinfoil remnants of lunch, she took out a crumpled paper and handed it to me. Ignoring the mess, I took it from her, making a mental note to clean out her backpack later. I had to pick my battles. I pulled out the chair and got her to sit down at the desk. I pushed her in, taking no chances of an escape, stood behind her and reached around to the crumpled homework sitting on the desk in front of her. She picked it up and started tossing it in the air. I caught it mid-flight and bent over her smallness to flatten the paper directly in front of her. Together we read the assignment.

Complete these three math review problems with what you learned today in class. This homework should take you no longer than fifteen minutes. Be sure to show me your work! —Mrs. Golden.

"Well, that shouldn't be hard for you. Where would you like to start?"

I could feel her fidgeting, squirming. Looking for a way out. I held strong, waiting.

"Mommy, I want to play a little more. I promise I will start as soon as I finish my dance."

Planting my feet firmly behind her, I jerked open the drawer a little too quickly in response, and took out a pencil, placing it in her chubby hands still sticky from her after school snack. I could feel the tension building in my shoulders. I breathed through it and stayed focused.

She accepted the pencil and looked up at my face hovering directly over her, absorbing my change in mood for a fleeting moment.

"It's okay, Mommy, we'll get it done. I just have to pee first."

She ducked under my arm and was gone before I knew it. I took the time to run downstairs to check on the twins. I could hear their giggles from the landing between floors; I stopped and peered into the living room. They were sitting just as I left them. I turned quickly and ran back upstairs, taking two steps at a time. Only ten minutes before their show ended, and then I'd have to leave Molly alone again while I set them up. I hated leaving them in front of the TV, but it was the best babysitter I had right now.

I saw she was back from the bathroom. I inhaled and reset my resolve. But, instead of starting the work we had just talked about, she was standing on top of the homework itself, which was already on top of the desk, with her tap shoes on, dancing.

I stood still, taking it all in for a split second. I tried to steady my voice, instead reminding myself to stay calm. My jaw tightened, holding back any words that would derail our progress. Instead, I stared directly at her. It barely seemed to register. Void of challenge to my authority, merely having fun, oblivious to any responsibility, she continued to dance, her tapping forcibly raising the tension in the room.

"Molly, get down. We have homework to do." I repeated the line over and over each time my voice rising in volume and lowering in pitch. Part of me envied her carefree nature. Part of me wanted to dress up like a fairy and twirl and dance and laugh with her. But more of me could not understand why she wasn't listening to me. The list of things I still had to get done ran through my mind on repeat.

Finish homework with Molly.
Get dinner ready.
Give all three kids baths.
Get all three kids ready for bed.
Read all three kids books and put them to sleep.

At this rate, we'd never get done. I could feel the panic growing.

Make lunches for tomorrow.
Clean up kitchen.

I clenched my teeth, clamping down hard, hoping I could keep from reaching my boiling point.

Clean up bathroom.
Collapse!!

No such luck. I shot across the room and grabbed her arm, tightening my grip until she stopped dancing.

"Ow... You're hurting me, Mommy."

I wish her words made me back off, but all they told me was it was working. I held on.

"Then get down now and let's start work," I said through clenched teeth.

I held on, helping her down from her stage and stood with my arms crossed next to her, daring her to get up again.

"Why are you angry, Mommy?"

Her innocence softened me a bit and I bent over her, trying

to slow my racing heart, reminding myself it was just homework. I was tired. This was happening every night. I worried if we couldn't get this homework done what would happen next year, or the year after that. My imagination ran wild picturing a broken future for my bright child. How would she ever get to college, never mind succeed there?

What was wrong with me?

Why couldn't I relax and enjoy my kids like everyone else?

I felt so alone. Like no one else was having these problems with kindergarten homework. She knew all her letters and numbers, was reading on her own, and could do simple math like make change, add, and subtract. She just couldn't stay focused. I had to be on her all the time. I knew she could do it and blamed myself for her difficulties. It was exhausting.

Downstairs I could hear the twins running around. I felt the pull. At two years old, they couldn't be left alone. I ran to the top of the steps and told them they could watch the next show and I'd be right down. I took a few deep breaths before I went back in her room. I rubbed her back and played with her hair as we both slowed down. *She's only five*, I reminded myself. *This will pass. Let's just get through tonight. Tomorrow will be better.*

"I'm not angry. I just know you can do your homework. I know it's easy for you, but you just have to sit and do it like Mrs. Golden asked. So, let's sit here until its done and then we can make dinner."

A few more starts and stops and we put the finishing touches on the homework. What was supposed to take *no more than fifteen minutes* had stretched into over an hour and a half. Total work time under ten minutes. I had to do better.

I knew something was not right and I was determined to figure it out and resolve it before she was aware and before she fell too far behind.

I wasted no time. During the summer between kindergarten and first grade, I took Molly to Dr. Karen Heller, a neuropsychologist, to run tests. The results, presented to us almost immediately, were conclusive. The test showed Molly was very bright. She had a high IQ. Then the doctor went on to explain, "Based on the results, I can confidently conclude she has attention deficit hyperactivity disorder (ADHD)."

I wasn't surprised. In fact, I was relieved. If she had a diagnosis that meant she was ill, a disease, something that was treatable and as her mom I could fix her. In years to come I would observe this reaction in too many friends with a diagnosed illness. The terror that comes from an unknown and the relief that somehow accompanies the diagnosis. When a clear path is suddenly laid out. Step one to step two to step three and so on. It was a challenge but one I rose to with the ferocity of a mama bear protecting its cub.

Things moved quickly then. I spent the rest of the summer understanding what I was up against. I felt like I was in a race against time. If I could get Molly all the resources she needed and make her better before her ADHD affected her performance in school, she'd never notice. Back then I believed she was still unaware of her differences. It wasn't until I was going through old papers for the purpose of writing this book that I found a line that stopped me dead in my tracks. In her report dated July 25, 2002, when Molly was six years, four months old, Dr. Heller wrote, "Molly made more than one comment about how stupid she thought she was..." I must have been so determined to find out what was wrong and fix her that I missed this critical piece of information. I don't know if we would have done anything differently, but knowing how she saw herself so early on was a red flag I wish I knew.

I became an expert in Pennsylvania education rights for children like Molly. I knew the school had up to sixteen weeks to test Molly on their own once I made a formal request and sent them Dr. Heller's findings. I didn't lose any time and sent Sharon Ryder, the principal of our elementary school, a letter in early August, hoping the clock could start immediately. Her response was even better than I expected. Sharon, a mom herself, responded with a promise to help, giving me the hope and encouragement I needed to forge on.

Mrs. Ryder was as good as her word, and during the quiet weeks of August, we wrote a 504 plan that gave Molly classroom support beginning in time for the start of first grade. Feeling confident that school was in good hands, I turned my attention to Molly's life outside of school.

I treated Molly's ADHD diagnosis like a degree I received before I took all the requisite classes and jumped into action to fill the gap. I devoured article after article noting that not everything fit but taking it all in anyway. I skimmed past the diagnosis sections, because we had that part in black and white from Dr. Heller, and moved right into treatments. If five treatments were recommended, I went on to research all five. Searching and searching for a cure.

I became a walking dictionary about ADHD and how to manage it, and our home became a living example. We had incentive charts taped on every surface imaginable. I pored over Oriental Trading catalogs. buying trinkets to entice all my children to follow the detailed routine I established.

I was determined to do everything in my power to fix her. We were a medical family. I believed in doctors. So I set out to find the experts. There was Margaret Fenton, the social skills expert whom Molly went to twice a week, learning everything from how to approach a group of kids at school to how to ask for something she wants. Eventually we stopped going because, for every situation practiced at Margaret's, Molly excelled. But in the real world she fell flat. I kept at it on my own, reviewing her social mishaps with her at the end of each day. I reasoned that like a child you tell fifty times not to touch an outlet, eventually she would learn to avoid the shock. The word *appropriate* became our mantra.

When I wasn't busy implementing one of the suggested treatments, social skills training class, creating a new behavior chart, or buying toys for incentives, I was reading and researching. I refused to wait to see if one thing was working before trying the next. In his book, *Outliers*, Malcolm Gladwell says it takes roughly 10,000 hours to become an expert at something, and I am confident I became an expert many times over in those early years.

I didn't let up. I didn't give myself a break. Order in my home was what I had control over. I matched every ounce of her inattention with a pound of attention to detail, to order, to plans that wouldn't allow for her to fail. I was spinning off in the opposite direction, barreling toward a vague ideal that I was sure was the answer to it all. I took lessons from my childhood, from our friends, and even from strangers on the street. They all seemed to have it so much more together than I, whose child was held just a little too tightly wherever we went. I never let go

When we left the house during the day I'd usher all three kids out the back door, down the patio steps, and into our minivan. Once they were safely buckled into their seats, distracted by a book or a video playing on the car VCR, I ran back into the house, taking the back steps two maybe three at a time.

I hurriedly cleaned up behind us. As if driven by the same motor that Molly created chaos, I recreated the calm before the storm. I returned toys to their baskets, put dirty dishes into the dishwasher, and wiped down all surfaces showing remnants from our morning routine. When I took a last look around surveying my handiwork, I could feel a sense of calm wash over me. I ran outside to the car and the waiting kids, this time locking the door behind me.

I knew it was unnecessary and a bit extreme, but I reasoned it was a coping mechanism that yielded positive results for everyone. Like straightening up your desk before leaving the office for the night makes it easier to start work the next day, my compulsion gave us a blank slate every time we came home. It was impossible to clean up when we were home—Molly was our very own tornado, always changing paths.

I also felt like I was doing it for Leo and Emily. I was painfully aware that so much of our life revolved around Molly's needs and they just got dragged along. With an eye toward *making memories*, I tried to make the chores in our life fun. I was a camp counselor for many summers, and I reasoned if I did it for fifteen six-year-olds, I should have no trouble with my three kids.

One weekend morning, I looked around the house between cleaning lady visits and saw an opportunity to make memories.

"Everyone downstairs, it's time for a family project."

All three kids tumbled into the kitchen still in their pajamas. Leo, in midsentence, came first, pushing his glasses back up his nose from where they had fallen in his hurry to be first. Emmy, always more cautious, but determined I know she heard me, was holding onto the railing and watching her three-year-old feet, repeating "Coming, Mommy" with each step. And then there was Molly. I could hear Howie urging her along and then herding her down the steps.

Leo stood in front of me impatiently shifting his weight from foot to foot. "What is it Mom, what's the project?" Emily attached herself to my hip echoing her brother's question. As I rubbed her back, she snuggled in close, almost pushing me over. I noted the nubby, worn feel of her feety pajamas. I could see the seams making dents in her shoulders—they were already too small. Time was passing so quickly. They were so full of life, ready for any adventure we created. I don't think they noticed yet how different their sister was, how she was shaping so much of what we did as a family.

Molly finally made her entrance, followed by Howie. I waited for her to stop moving, and with Emily still attached, I bent down and looked Molly straight in the eye but spoke to everyone.

"We're all going to clean up together!"

They were too young to protest or even throw me an eyeroll. I explained that there were cleaning jobs written on tokens in the jar and everyone was to pick one. Once you finished, you picked another one. Once everything was done you got to pick a toy from the treat jar for each token you had.

I glanced up at Howie. "You too?"

"Sure," he said, barely suppressing a laugh. "It will be fun."

And for the next forty-five minutes or so, it was.

We went to see a developmental pediatrician, Dr. Donna Ferracci. I immediately felt my shoulders relax as Molly ran off to one of the many play areas around the waiting room. This room was set up for children like Molly. Multiple play centers, all in view of a central seating area. For once I felt safe talking to the receptionist without needing eyes in the back of my head.

"For Molly Ross?"

I looked up and then down. I was barely done filling out the lengthy health and developmental history forms when we were called. I gathered everything and hurried after Molly and Howie. The three of us fit comfortably in the exam room with Dr. Ferracci, a no-nonsense woman whose eyes followed Molly's every move as she explored the room while we shared our story.

"Are you interested in medicine?"

Molly sat up straight, still holding the blood pressure cuff she had put around her arm and announced proudly. "Yes. My daddy is a doctor. He's a surgeon."

"Well, do you know how to take a pill? If I give your mom medicine to help you focus, you will need to take one a day."

"I can do it," Molly promised without hesitation, her head bobbing for emphasis.

As they discussed how to take a pill and listening to what to expect as we tried different medications, I let hope bloom and for a few minutes fantasized what our family life could be like if Molly didn't always take center stage. If I could take my eyes off her for just a minute without someone getting my attention to get control of her.

Dr. Ferracci had a sample of Metadate in her office and worked with Molly to get her first pill down. After a few tries…success!

Dr. Ferracci gave me our marching orders, now speaking as if Molly weren't in earshot.

"You should notice a change shortly. It won't always be so easy, and she has to be consistent. Maybe have a toy she really wants ready after she takes it successfully at home the first time? Keep track of her behavior and anything you notice."

I listened, planning to order Kit, the American Girl Doll Molly wanted, as soon as I had a free moment.

We left Dr. Ferracci with a prescription in hand and a follow-up appointment scheduled.

We picked up Leo and Emily and headed to our favorite pizza place, Peace A Pizza, for lunch. Howie was paying for the food while I brought back crayons and coloring books. It's funny how you don't notice the absence of things, so it took a few moments to register but when it did, I ran to Howie, grabbed his hand, and led him back to the kids, signaling him to be quiet. Together, we stood there glowing as if our kids were doing something miraculous, and to us they were. Leo, Emily, and…Molly were sitting quietly, focused on their coloring, at the pint-sized tables in the back of the restaurant.

I thought this medication was the answer, and it helped many things over the years, but seeing Molly today with thoughts of harming herself, I wondered if there was more going on than the ADHD. I had spent years trying to fix and get ahead of the problem, but here I was responding to a phone call that seemed destined to change everything. I'd give anything to be watching her dancing on her homework or climbing the steps painted purple rather than curled in a ball looking so lost. What did I miss? Another checklist started going off in my head.

Had she been sleeping?

Eating?

In her room more than usual?

Stop that! I scolded myself silently. It wouldn't help her now.

With Molly listening, Mrs. Ellicot continued answering my questions as if she had been in the car with me. It seemed the threat of failing classes triggered Molly's retreat, hands raised in surrender to the workload that had become too overwhelming. It was simple, even understandable. It was the leap she too readily made from giving up at school to giving up at life that was terrifying.

I understood where we had to go next. A threat, even a consideration of suicide, required a psychiatric evaluation and an *all clear* before returning to school. Still feeling like this was all happening to someone else, I dug deep to remain calm for Molly, finding some comfort knowing the next steps were laid out for us.

I let the counselor finish, managed to eke out a thank you past the lump in my throat, and scooped Molly up. We drove the short two miles to the local emergency room in silence except for a quick phone call to Howie, who luckily worked at the same hospital, to meet us when we got there. I stared at the road in front of me, trying not to think past getting to the hospital safely. Howie would be there. I wasn't in this alone. Molly moved quickly through admissions and was sent to the children's wing for observation. She livened up at all the attention and was more than willing to explain what she was upset about. While she continued to talk to the nurses, all of whom were obviously taken by her, the ER pediatric psych attending took us into another room.

Once there, he began an exhausting session gathering family history. A sense of detachment came over me as we told him everything we knew about Molly's birth parents. Like a robot I poured out all we know, which was more than many in our position. With each piece of information, I felt like I was passing the baton. Surely, he would fix her. We explained the psychologist who evaluated the birth parents prior to the adoption suspected they both had borderline personality disorder *(BPD)* but couldn't make a full diagnosis. He noted BPD on Molly's chart, but as borderline is considered an adult disease, not diagnosed until at least eighteen, that is where it remained.

After a while it all just sounded like noise. A maternal pull drew me to the room next door. Molly looked so small in the hospital bed. Still believing I could protect her from whatever we were up against, I snuggled in right beside her and wrapped my arms around her tiny frame.

I hugged her tight and kissed the top of her head. We lay there in silence, and despite all that was going on, I felt my eyes grow heavy. It had already been a long day. I wondered what time it was. As I glanced at my watch, I sat up and snapped back to reality. One of us had to pick Leo and Emily up from school, and whoever that was had to tell them where their sister was and why.

An internal tug of war began. I wanted, no I needed, to be in two places. I didn't want to leave Molly, but I also needed to be the one to explain to the twins.

I got to the school just as the doors opened, marking the end of what was just another day to everyone else. Watching the scene unfold, I felt like was going through the motions of a life that belonged to someone else. While I felt like an imposter, Leo and Emily didn't notice and thought I was the same mom they kissed goodbye six hours earlier. Emily hopped up first, stopping for a peck on my cheek before jumping up on her bucket seat in the second row, her backpack zippered up over her purple jacket, full of smiles and an infectious love for life. Leo followed, his glasses perched halfway down his nose as he tried to hold his loose papers, his open backpack offering an easy but overlooked solution. He was already mid-sentence telling me about his day, perhaps trying to get a verbal jump on his sister but forgetting that I need to be in earshot to hear the whole story. As the familiar scene unfolded in the rearview mirror, I took a mental snapshot realizing nothing was or would be the same again.

There was no choice but to tell the twins. I recently learned it was futile trying to protect them from what was going on in their own home. Just a few weeks earlier, Leo's disorganization began affecting his grades and I was trying to work with him. Anything I suggested was met with an eyeroll and a placating nod. It had nothing to do with the level or the amount of work, much of the time he even had the work completed but failed to hand it in. The zeros were piling up. Finally, I suggested a tutor specializing in organizing strategies. The tears wet the inside of his glasses before I even finished, and I suddenly understood.

"Are you afraid there's something wrong with you if I get you a tutor?"

"Yes," he said, "like Molly."

I knew that if he was old enough to make that connection, he, as well as Emily, was old enough to hear the truth. While difficult, it was far better than leaving them to fill in their suspicions with fiction or fantasy.

We drove home, with me nodding in all the right places even as I wondered what was going on at the hospital. I tried to plan what I would say but only tripped over my own words and had made no progress by the time the garage door opened.

Still chatting about their days, they ran inside and wiggled out of their backpacks, stepping over them and the jackets that followed.

"Grab a snack and meet me on the couch," I yelled after them.

They both stopped mid-sentence, turned to look at me and then each other. They never had snacks on the couch. They did as I asked without question but moved much slower than usual, like they were avoiding what was coming. I sat at the end of the couch facing them, noting their legs still didn't touch the ground. They were so little, and what I had to talk to them about was so big. Too big. All day I had felt like things would never be the same and this was the point of no return. I knew there was no way out but forward. I stopped thinking, took a deep breath, and ripped off the band-aid.

"Molly is in the hospital. She is okay, but she had some bad thoughts about hurting herself, so the doctors are going to talk to her until she feels better."

And there it was. We crossed the threshold into a reality I had been avoiding for years. My attempts to shield, protect, fix, even medicate Molly just covering up something deeper that was brewing inside of her. Having ADHD was fairly common. Anything more than that put us in a different category entirely.

I didn't realize the critical turning point this discussion was in Leo and Emily's emotional, personal, and even professional paths. All I saw were two children confused and scared and wanting to know that all would be okay. I went ahead and assured them even though I had no business doing so. We talked about how they could help when Molly came home. How they could be extra nice, and more patient even when she did something that annoyed them or that was inappropriate, a common word in our household. It seemed so simple as we sat there on the couch. I was still super mom with powers to fix everything. I let them have that fantasy for as long as it held.

We headed to the hospital in silence. Once they saw Molly in her room, they seemed to come alive again. Molly was her usual chatty self, enjoying the attention and impressing the docs with her medical knowledge. As became a familiar pattern, these crises pass. With each one we learned something, we regrouped, and we moved on. Sometimes we moved forward, but sometimes we just moved on in the same place we were before. After this one, our first hospitalization, we moved on and forward. Things changed. Some were scary, like locking away knives and medication. Others were laying the foundation for the new status quo *(I hate the word normal)*, like finding a therapist, a psychiatrist, telling our family and friends, and involving the school and teachers. For the moment, we were focused on taking our fingers off the trigger: overdue work assignments, feelings of isolation, and feelings of failure both academically and socially. But we weren't fooling ourselves anymore. This wasn't a single occurrence, but a fork in our road. We needed to prepare for what lay ahead, and giving air to what was really going on in our home laid the groundwork to do just that.

We took her home that night. Howie and I armed with hospital directives and an outpatient plan. The kids, Molly included, mostly concerned with what we were eating for dinner. We picked up takeout, and over disposable containers and cans of soda, we talked about what had happened. It was the first of many *family meetings*. This one far from the contentious ones to come, more like teammates regrouping after a rough game. I remember finding it hard to focus, trying to find comfort knowing she was safe in our house, and knowing for the moment we all were.

CHAPTER SIX

Warrior One

"Inhale, sweep your arms up overhead. Swan dive forward. Inhale halfway up. Exhale. Release. Inhale, place hands on floor, and step one foot back and then the other. Lift your hips up. Welcome to your first downward dog of the day."

It was a beautiful day in Meadowridge Park. The green space in the middle of town was full of flower buds begging to open. Their promise usually made me feel hopeful but was lost on me today. Instead, I was intently focused on my phone, completely out of sync with my surroundings.

There were ten people signed up for the run/yoga class I was teaching for the Jersey Shore Tri-Gals, a group of women founded by my closest friends, that trained together for triathlons. I created today's class to share the mind/body benefits of yoga for runners.

When we first moved to Fair Haven, I waited until the kids and Howie were settled in their new schools and job respectively and most of the boxes were unpacked before I took out the card my yoga teacher from Philadelphia handed me after my last class. Blue Moon Yoga was only a ten-minute drive from our new home, and I started classes whenever I could sneak one in. I liked the people, but more than that I liked having a regular practice. Whatever was happening at home didn't make its way onto my mat. Since I began practicing about two years earlier, I found myself treasuring my time on the mat, and the more I practiced yoga the more I understood and embraced yogic beliefs on and off my mat. I even dressed the part, purchasing my first set of mala beads and wearing them proudly out on a Saturday night.

Yoga helped me find balance in what had become a very unbalanced life. Driven so often by the needs of the kids and even Howie, I rarely thought about, never mind tended to, my own needs. I was starting to forget what they even were. I wanted to take it to the next level and share what I found to be a way to find peace in the growing chaos. Becoming a yoga instructor was a big commitment so before I brought it up with Howie, I did what I do best. I made a list:

Pros
A chance to share my newest coping skill—a way to find peace in chaos
A chance to be stable and strong for my family
A chance to feel successful in at least one part of my life
A chance to stay in good shape
A chance to contribute financially
A chance to be someone besides a mother and a wife
And I love the clothes!

Cons
Cost of Teacher Training
Time away from the family

Armed with my list, I spit it out one night when Howie and I had a quiet moment.

"I'd like to take the yoga teacher training at Blue Moon Yoga. It's a big commitment—200 hours of class time—mostly weekends over six months. I'd also have to take three to four classes a week. Of course, I could do those while the kids are at school. And it's not cheap—but then I'd be certified to teach!"

He smiled and, without missing a beat, assured me we'd make it work.

And we did. It wasn't always as easy as he promised. I came home to a lot of messes during those weekends—both ones left for me to clean up with a sponge and ones waiting for me to mediate, negotiate, or dole out punishments for.

But it was worth it. Each weekend was like a mini vacation. I loved learning. What a gift after years of wondering if my brain still worked!

The eight-hour days flew by. Our class of six soon felt like family, sharing intimate details of the hows and whys we all found yoga. Each day was a mix of classroom learning and movement. We broke down each pose, later putting them back together during classes we taught to each other. I blossomed like a lotus flower, a popular symbol of rebirth in many yoga studios, during those months. Before long I tossed my notes, put on my mala beads, and quieted the butterflies in my stomach. When I was in front of a class, I was a yoga teacher and soon enough a studio owner, and at least to my students, I wasn't "poor Molly's mom."

I graduated in a small ceremony with my family in attendance and began teaching at an older studio about a half mile from my house. I taught private lessons before the kids woke up, morning classes while they were at school, and a few in the evening that were harder to juggle. When the opportunity arose to take over the studio, I jumped at it, sure I could transform it from a sleepy small-town studio to a Jersey Shore icon.

Fair Haven Yoga was all mine, and I flourished in the next few months. I redesigned the studio to create a more serene, welcoming space. I painted the walls a muted blue, added bamboo flooring and room dividers. I purchased new mats and even added lavender scented eye pillows for students to end class with. I hired new teachers, taught eight to ten classes a week myself, and spent every free moment thinking of ways to build traffic. Vino and vinyasa on Friday nights, couples' yoga, teen and kids' classes, chair yoga, even birthday parties on the weekend. Slowly they came.

What I didn't anticipate was the constant pulling between home and work. Some days I was stretched so thin I felt like saltwater taffy. The studio and our house were less than a mile apart, but I couldn't seem to bridge the gap. Howie pitched in when he could, but his job still came first. I was my own boss, and my earnings were still in the red of a new business.

I thought owning the studio would help, and in many ways it did. It gave Molly a place to work, something to do and build her resume, while I could keep an eye on her and hope the smells of sage and the serene surroundings would somehow do their magic. But over time the studio became more of a drain. Molly spent more time in and out of the hospital. Each time I left her at an inpatient facility the sun rose the next morning, and I managed to put on the face of a functioning adult and go on with my day.

But the day came when I knew I had to close the studio. It wasn't the first time Molly was hospitalized, but her illness was becoming more demanding as we searched for a diagnosis that fit, treatments that worked, and fought for moments of normalcy in between it all. Balancing home and work was becoming impossible, and I felt like I was failing at both. Something had to give *soon*.

Even though we had been through it all before, it never got any easier when Molly was an in-patient. This time was no different. I moved through the morning as if in a trance, allowing Charley, our yellow lab, to lick any tears from my face before my feet hit the floor. Driven by routine, my hands reached for my black yoga pants and purple tank top. I wrapped myself in the coziest cardigan I could find as if the chenille could protect me from the rest of my life. I knew I'd be barefoot once I got to work but still put on my furry slippers until I left. None of it warmed the chill that had settled in my bones when I left the hospital the night before.

I opened the doors to the twins' bedrooms enough to keep my puffy eyes in the early morning shadows while letting in the forced lilt in my voice.

"Time to wake up, Emily."

"Time to wake up, Leo."

Their grunts assured me they were awake before I headed downstairs. This part was easy. I moved around the kitchen, preparing breakfast, enjoying the familiarity of the routine. I grabbed the bread from the counter and put two pieces in the toaster oven. While that was cooking, I filled the cup with the ingredients I had long perfected for Emily's morning smoothie. Half a banana, some sun nut butter, milk, protein powder, a little spinach, and four ice cubes. While I reached into the refrigerator for the spinach and milk, I grabbed the cream cheese knowing it would top Leo's toast. He'd also finish the banana and maybe a yogurt. I tightened the cover on the smoothie cup and turned it upside down, twisting it into the Ninja until I heard the satisfying click followed immediately by grinding signaling success.

I prepared my smile with as much precision as the smoothie

and was ready when they came downstairs. I tried to balance my cheeriness with the heaviness they were surely feeling.

"How are you guys feeling this morning?"

Neither of them answered right away, instead they searched my face for answers that I didn't have. I tried to reassure them so they could go on with their day.

"She'll be okay. She's in a safe place. After I teach my classes, I'm going to head over for visiting hours. Do either of you want to come?" I held my breath.

Leo shook his head no right away and Emily followed.

I sighed. It was better this way. Routine. Normalcy. It was the best way I could think to protect them.

I probably held on a little too long before they left to start their days at middle school, but they let me. I guess we all needed it.

As I drove to the studio, I let myself think about what was going on. Alone in the car with my thoughts, the tears fell, and I resisted the urge to call anyone, instead trying to gather myself before I faced the day. I thought about how excited I was to open Fair Haven Yoga. I loved being part of the community, building a business, having something that was all my own. On days like this, however, I could barely remember the draw and only felt the drain. It took all I had to get Leo and Emily to school, and I needed to have something left for my visit with Molly.

My hand shook as I tried to fit the key into the lock. The scent of sage from last night's classes didn't have its usual effect. I turned the heat up as high as I could and began going about my day.

I turned on the lights and glanced at the pictures that adorned the wall. A tree of life, a hand drawn *ohm,* and a picture of my studio, all generously gifted to me by a local artist and friend. Above my desk was a membership certificate from the Fair Haven Business Association. I reached under my desk to find the slippers I kept for cold days. I needed them today.

I opened the doors connecting the office to the studio and walked in, thankful for the grippies on the slippers. I picked up the signup sheet for the day's classes. Six people. A good number. Too few students and I'd feel responsible for ongoing conversation. Too many would feel overwhelming right now. Before I put down the schedule, I glanced at the name of the class I was to teach in fifteen minutes.

YOGA FOR MENTAL WELL-BEING.

I stared like I was seeing it for the first time. I shouldn't be shocked. I made the schedule and created the class. But on this day the irony struck me as cruel, and I sank to the floor under the weight of all I was carrying.

How could I possibly teach a class on mental well-being when I was barely holding on by a thread?

I already knew the answer. It was the same answer to how I moved around much of my life when Molly was in crisis. I did what I had to do.

I laid out the mats and realized I had a few minutes before anyone would arrive. While I couldn't give myself more quiet time, I could make the most of what I had. I sat down cross legged on the closest mat, closed my eyes, and slipped almost immediately into a deep meditative state. As the familiar warmth surrounded me, my heart slowed, and a smile appeared that was as real as the tears that drizzled down my cheeks. I gave myself a quick hug and stood up, as ready as I'd ever be.

And as the students arrived, I smiled and greeted them. They didn't notice the effort it took or the fact my voice sounded foreign as I got it around the lump that had re-emerged in my throat. They came for a yoga class on mental well-being and that is what I gave them.

Shortly after that class, I closed the studio but was still

teaching sporadically to groups such as the Tri Gals locally. It worked better for the unpredictability of my life.

I picked this day to teach in the park carefully. Because it was a Tuesday, the kids were at school, freeing me up to volunteer my time. I hadn't planned for being caught in the aftermath of another hospitalization. I don't remember what precipitated this one, only that it was part of a growing number of confrontations and crises that were becoming more and more difficult to resolve without intervention. Each one took so much out of me, but I had made a commitment and here I was. Luckily teaching was routine, and I quickly got down to business.

My yoga voice came naturally, and we moved easily through a series of sun salutations. Each time we came back to a plank I glanced down at my phone. Still no call. I was waiting for Dr. Ellman, a therapist recommended by Dr. Franklin, the psychiatrist assigned to her by the hospital.

We met Dr. Franklin yesterday. Her office was a playground to Molly—decorated in hundreds of troll dolls. While we waited, Molly busied herself with the trolls while I split my time between tapping my feet, wondering if Molly was making too big of a mess, and hoping this doctor could help.

Dr. Franklin was a small, round woman with teeth as bright as the smile she gave us.

"I see you like my troll collection," she said warmly with a hint of amusement in her tone.

Her attention stayed with Molly, referring to me only as *Mom* and only on occasion.

"Molly, let's talk for a bit. Why don't you sit down, and you can tell me why you're here. Is that okay with you, Mom?"

I nodded and watched the rest unfold. As the two of them talked it was clear Dr. Franklin knew what she was doing.

She listened to Molly but was no pushover. She kept digging, obviously trying to get to know her patient.

"But you don't actually want to hurt yourself, so why do you keep threatening to do so?"

As they moved past the most current episode and on to troubles at school, with friends, and at home, it was clear Dr. Franklin understood Molly. I stopped tapping my feet and instead found myself nodding along in agreement.

"It sounds to me, Miss Molly, that you have a lot of things you are unhappy about but need some help in fixing them..."

We both nodded emphatically. As we wrapped up, Dr. Franklin prescribed new meds to address Molly's growing list of complaints of anxiety, anger, and depression that the old meds didn't seem to be helping, and talked about new strategies Molly should try. She continued to speak directly to Molly, getting her buy-in with each step.

"So, you will take these new meds every day and then tell me how they make you feel. I want it all. The good, the bad, and the ugly. And you're going to work with Mom to make lists of what you have to do and break them down and give yourself small rewards each time you do something. Like a half hour of television, or time on your computer. Right, Miss Molly?"

While I wasn't included in much of the conversation, I felt like I had found an ally. As Molly ran out of the room ahead of us, Dr. Franklin looked up at me, slightly out of breath from standing up, and said, "She's going to be okay...but it will be a bumpy road."

As a psychiatrist, Dr. Franklin was primarily responsible for prescribing Molly's meds. She recommended Dr. Ellman as a therapist. I called and left a message on our way home that night.

Still no sign of Dr. Ellman by the time we finished out last sun salutation, so I laid out the plans for our run and how to benefit from the yoga/running combination.

"One time around the figure eight is one mile. We are going to run around once and meet back here to stretch and then repeat with intervals for the second time. After that we'll meet back for a cool down. Try to keep your mind as clear on the run as you did during yoga and remember to use the breathing we just practiced."

I led the group and Pam, President of the JSTG and a close friend, followed. Pam and I talked all the time, and I knew she had my back today and every day. As I took off at a quicker pace than usual, I relished the quiet time away from the group. I always ran faster during times of stress as if I could outrun my problems. Today I flew.

Just as I returned to our circle of empty yoga mats, my phone rang. I stepped to the other side of the dirt figure eight, and with barely a glance Pam knew it was the call I was waiting for. Without missing a beat, she took over the lead for the second mile, giving me the privacy and time I needed.

"Hello?" I answered the phone, hopeful.

"Hello, this is Dr. Ellman. I'm returning your call."

There was something in his voice that touched me immediately. The gravelly tone told me he had experience. And the time he took sharing his thoughts after I summarized the past fourteen years told me he was really listening. I was practiced in telling my story to doctors and sped through it. I knew much of it would come up again later and didn't want to invest too much until I knew if this was a good match. But this time, I immediately felt it was right.

He must have agreed.

"I'd like the chance to meet Molly and talk. How is tomorrow?"

We got down to business and set up an appointment at his

Red Bank office for the next day after school. He gave me the address and we said goodbye.

As I walked back to the dirt track, the promise of springtime in the park finally touched me. I felt hope blossoming in my chest like the flowers around me. Dr. Ellman had lightened my load just a little bit. I smiled to myself—a real smile—and took off.

CHAPTER SEVEN

A Lot on the Line

"Hello?"
"Hi, Stacy, it's Dad. You have a baby brother!"

The call we had been waiting for. I beat Gramps to the black rotary phone sitting at a desk in the hallway right outside the kitchen.

September 12, 1971.

The day I became a big sister. I was almost five and ready for the responsibility. I'd listened to everyone telling me how my little brother *(or sister)* was going to look up to me and think I was the greatest thing in the world. That was a lot to live up to. I had it all planned. We would be best friends. We'd have a secret language, maybe even find a secret spot in our apartment just for us. He or she *(I couldn't wait to find out!)* would follow me around, and I was going to take such good care of him *(or her)*. My mom and dad would be so proud of me and my grandparents too! They always told me it was important to make my parents proud. I never wanted them to roll their eyes or get angry at me the way they did with my cousins, Andrew and Jon, when they came to visit. Jon didn't always listen and sometimes Andrew and Jon punched each other. When Nana, who wasn't much taller than my cousins already, had had enough, Gramps would "step in." He was usually always happy and laughed at us as we ran around their house. But when he got angry, he seemed so much bigger and pointed his finger at the boys telling them to "stop it right now." He never had to be that way with me. No one would need to tell me to stop anything when I had my own brother *(or sister)*. I was going to be the best big sister ever!

I was practicing being the best big sister that day. My mom, dad, and Nana were at the hospital waiting for the baby. I was home with Gramps. Nana told me Gramps needed me to keep him company, and Gramps told me he needed help making lunch since Nana always did it.

"I can do it!" I told them. They promised they'd call as soon as there was any "news." That's grown-up talk for the baby being born.

Gramps' favorite was peanut butter and banana sandwiches. I loved them too, especially when I was with him. I volunteered to make them all by myself! Gramps said he'd watch from his big blue chair in the living room, but he wasn't even looking at me. He was watching the ball game on the little white TV. He kept moving around the antennas and yelling angry words when the picture looked like snow or he didn't like something one of his guys did. He wasn't watching me at all. He knew he didn't have to!

I took the jar of peanut butter out of the metal pantry standing in the corner of the kitchen. I knew to be careful not to climb on it since Jon tipped the whole thing over last Thanksgiving. Everyone was so angry! I pulled a wooden chair from the table and stood on it to reach the jar. Then I carefully got down, balancing the jar in my hands, put it on the table, and moved the chair back where it belonged. I didn't forget to close the pantry either. Next, I took white bread and a banana off the counter where Nana leaves them. Last I found the paper plates and a knife to spread. I knew to take the butter knife since it was safest like Gramps said.

With all the ingredients in front of me I began preparing lunch for Gramps and me. I took out two paper plates and four pieces of bread. Then I carefully opened the jar of peanut butter. It was hard to get my hand around the top, but I tried really, really hard and finally the top turned. Next, I dipped the knife deep into the jar covering the whole knife and coming up with enough peanut butter for both of us. I carefully spread it out like I watched Nana do many times before. First on one piece of Gramp's bread, then on mine, careful to split it equally. I peeled the waiting banana and used the knife to cut circles, sticking them into the peanut butter covered bread. All that was left was to cover the peanut butter and banana with the other piece of white bread. My stomach was growling, and I couldn't wait to show Gramps I could make him lunch as good as Nana.

So, we were ready and waiting when the phone rang. When I heard the news, I dropped the phone and turned to Gramps.

"It's a brother!" I yelled, now standing on the desk chair, wrapped in the phone cord.

He laughed and took the phone for more "details." But I didn't need to know anymore. I had a brother!

I listened to them make plans for when we could meet my brother. I was jumping up and down asking more questions while he was talking.

"What's his name? When can we meet him? Where's Mommy? Tell them about the sandwiches I made!"

"Well Stacy and I are about to eat what I bet are the best

peanut butter and banana sandwiches I ever had and then we'll drive over. She's taking very good care of me!"

I started smiling so big I couldn't even talk anymore. I didn't know which I was more excited about at that moment, making Gramps lunch or the baby brother I was going to meet afterwards. I bounced back to the kitchen and put the finishing touches on our sandwiches.

Lunch is served!

* * *

After Molly left Riverview Medical Center that first time, things were never the same for me. I never heard the phone ring quite the same way again. What used to be an invitation became a taunt, a threat, "Answer me…I dare you."

I knew that what could be on the other end of the phone could very well be the next crisis. I never stopped wondering, waiting for it to happen all over again.

Some might say in doing so I missed a lot of the good things. That it was a lot of energy to waste when all that worry wouldn't stop those crises. And they would be right. I know that now. I knew it before. But it was this middle part, when I was so deep in the thick of it that I couldn't see my way out.

I wasn't wrong. I wanted the fairytale. I wanted to curl up in my pink bedroom with my pink comforter and my pink shag rug, on my telephone talking for hours about school, boys, gossip. Lighter times. Simpler times.

But now, every phone call was just an inhale as I waited for the other shoe to drop. And drop they did. They came in the form of phone calls, emails, and even in-person meetings.

There was the phone call telling me Molly was fired from her job as a counselor-in-training at Sand Dollar Day Camp after yelling at her bus driver in front of a bus full of campers.

There was the phone call threatening to throw Molly out

of summer camp for *inappropriate behavior* in the dining room with her boyfriend.

There were the almost daily emails from teachers warning me that Molly's zeros for missed assignments and missed classes put her in danger of failing.

There were the phone calls from the school guidance counselor telling me the same.

There was the phone call from her friend Amy's parents telling me we needed to pick up Molly from their home as she, at sixteen, was behaving seductively with their thirteen-year-old son.

Each one a punch in my gut, leaving me breathless.

Like a boxer I continued to get up, but round after round the blows added up and the idea to just stay down for the count, at times, sounded appealing.

I started to fantasize what it would feel like if I could escape the almost daily onslaught.

What if I ran away?

I tried to take breaks. I knew the importance of self-care and I had begun building a healthy coping toolbox. I practiced yoga, tried to take time for myself with friends, and Howie and I stayed committed to our date nights.

And then there was running.

I started running during my senior year in college. I'd leave our ground floor apartment at the top of the hill in Collegetown, letting the screen door slam behind me as I walked down the famous hills of Ithaca until I reached the flatter route I mapped out for myself. As I ran through fraternity row, I could see the Ivy League buildings in all their glory dotting campus above me, and if I peeked between houses adorned with Greek letters, I could just make out Cayuga Lake far below. The view never got old, and as I ran my three miles day after day, I fell more in love with my home away from home. But I also started to fall in love with my time on the pavement.

As I've gotten older, it's harder to get started, those first few steps as shockingly painful as stepping into an ice filled tub. I expect it and, like a train picking up steam, so do I as I work out the morning creakiness and get my natural juices flowing. Some days it takes a while to warm up and I feel every bit of my fifty-five years. The harshness of the pavement reverberating up my legs giving my sciatica something to complain about. Other days I immediately feel like I'm flying. My legs light, each step carrying me, and I get to be a passenger. It's those days that keep me coming back for more.

Many things have changed since those early days of running. I had several careers, married, and raised three children. At each stage I kept running.

When Molly's illness took center stage, running was often my sanctuary. I'd head outside and let my feet carry me away from whatever conflict was brewing at home. When the proverbial shoes dropped, I put my running shoes on. My pace often matched the crisis, picking up speed as I replayed difficult scenes in my head. On the morning after Molly's first hospitalization, I waited until the twins left for school, resisting the pull of my bed, and headed outside, phone in my lap belt just in case. My legs felt like lead from lack of sleep, and I wondered if I'd be able to breathe through the lump lodged in my throat. I walked for a bit, and instinctively my feet took over. First a slow jog. The wind starting to work its magic clearing out the dark thoughts. A little faster, drying the tears running down my cheeks. And then, quite unexpectedly, my mouth began to curl in an unfamiliar shape. I was smiling.

Without realizing it I had found my biggest coping skill. A meditation in movement.

But it seemed I couldn't outrun the growing storm in my

own home. Like a hurricane it gathered strength over the years, piling up debris in its path. Even though running and other coping skills gave me well needed breaks, it got to be that stepping away was barely worth it for the mess that was waiting for me when I got back. I began to run only if I was sure all was quiet, sometimes watching the time I'd set aside get shorter and shorter as I made phone calls, cleaned up, or answered emails. Sometimes I missed them all together.

The phone calls continued, and I was powerless to do anything but answer them and deal with the aftermath. It seemed the life I dreamt of was slipping away. And then there was the added pain of the phone calls I had to make to others further exposing an already painful wound.

"Mom, I lost her. I tried so hard, but I failed. They're taking her away and I don't know if she's ever coming back."

It all came out in a rush of words. I was screaming, crying, and gasping for air like a drowning victim desperate for a lifeline. At forty-seven years old, I still hoped my parents could save me.

My mom and dad knew I had taken Molly to the emergency room again after her guidance counselor at Windward High School called to tell me Molly didn't feel safe with herself. She was almost seventeen years old and this was by no means the first time I'd gotten that call, but this time was different. This time, when I picked her up at school, she wouldn't look at me. Her face was flat, stoic, almost zombie-like. When I approached her, she turned on me like a bear woken from hibernation, making actual grunting noises and speaking in a voice that was deep and threatening, like it was coming from someone else.

"Don't come near me, Stacy."

For the first time I was truly afraid of my own daughter.

She agreed to leave with me but kept her distance. We rode

in the car like two strangers. She wouldn't engage. She growled like an animal warning me when I tried to speak to her.

I took her to the emergency room at our local hospital, even though I knew she couldn't stay there. They didn't have a pediatric psych unit, but I thought she'd be released or transferred locally like every other time. I was caught off guard when they recommended transfer to a longer term psychiatric hospital that was better equipped to deal with her and help us figure out the next steps.

I had to leave her there as they arranged transportation. She still wouldn't look at me and I still didn't understand why. The school claimed to have no idea either, and after all these years I still don't know why Molly shut down. What sticks out more from that day is when she looked right through me and told the ER doctors she didn't want to live at home anymore.

I held it all together, absorbing blow after blow. I stayed in the corner, observing, not trusting my voice. When asked, I managed to squeak out answers to the doctors' questions.

"Yes, please transfer her where you think best."

"We need to find out what is going on."

"No, nothing specific happened, I don't know why she won't talk to me."

"If she doesn't want to live with us, we'll figure it out."

"No, I don't think there are any drugs involved."

It wasn't until I left the hospital without her that it hit me. I lost her. No matter how hard I worked, no matter how hard I tried, no matter how much I loved and mothered her, this still fully undiagnosed illness was fighting me every step of the way.

I didn't know what to do. I was beaten. Feeling like a façade of a mom, a failure of a daughter, a farce of a yoga practitioner, I could not see a way out. By the time I hung up with my parents, they were packing and booking flights. For once I didn't argue.

When I got back to the hospital with Leo and Emily, Molly seemed better. She was happy to see the twins but still wouldn't look at me or Howie.

I couldn't help but feel judged by the doctor. He asked us again if we knew why Molly didn't want to come home.

"Did something happen?"

"Is there a lot of fighting in your house?"

"Is she afraid of something, or either one of you?"

NO!

NO!!

NO!!!

Sometimes it's just easier to be angry.

With no answers, he repeated to both of us what he had explained earlier. Molly would be transferred by ambulance to Dryden Clinic because 1) she had a plan to harm herself and 2) she did not want to come home.

The next morning, I cried the whole way in the car with my parents following the ambulance, any pretense of composure long shed. It was probably better Molly still wouldn't look at me when they helped her out, her arms immobile from the straitjacket they put her in for the ride. We watched her go into the building. Dryden Clinic was a cold looking brick building set in sparse surroundings. It looked as isolated and lonely on the outside as I was sure many of its inhabitants felt on the inside. We just stood on the gravel driveway staring, as a large white door, looking more like the entrance to a meat locker than a care facility, slammed behind Molly. Left alone in the stillness, we didn't know what to do next. We didn't have to wait long. A nurse called to us from the front entrance.

"Are you here for Molly Ross?"

I nodded, and as if in a dream, followed her through the empty waiting area and into a sterile office where, with barely a word, she pointed to the necessary paperwork before leaving me alone. I tried to focus, but my hands were shaking so badly the insurance numbers I wrote on those tiny lines were barely legible. She didn't seem to notice, instead trading me the intake forms for a sheet of paper containing nothing more than visiting hours and a promise a doctor would call later with an update.

We went back to our house and ordered something for dinner. My brother drove down after work and while I was glad to see him, I felt like I was on the outside of my life watching a scene from an afterschool special, a TV drama, or even *Ordinary People*.

But this wasn't a TV show. This was my real life, and I had no choice but to wait. I concentrated on making sure I was breathing and that in itself felt like an Olympic event. The mood was somber. No one knew what to say. I usually led the conversation, but I was running on empty. It was all so hard. The wondering, the waiting, the palpable sadness blanketing the house.

Leo threw me a life preserver that night and I don't know if he knows that to this day. The mailman showed up with a letter from Communications High School and even though he wasn't home I peeked. I suspected it was good news and grabbed at the chance like a refugee stumbling into camp and being offered a hot meal.

I was right!

Communications High School was one of five county academies with a tough application process that looked at a combination of grades, recommendations, and an admissions test. Only one to two students were accepted from each area high school every year.

He got in! I let out a yell so full of emotion—so happy to be able to be happy—to prove to everyone and myself that we had a good life, that Molly's illness was just part of it.

Of course, then I had to close the envelope and make everyone promise to keep quiet until he opened it himself a little while later. But it was just what I needed to get through the night.

A faceless, nameless doctor did call from Dryden. There was no one specific assigned to Molly and the information we were given was as vague as my memories of the call itself. I learned she was safe, was being evaluated, was under 24-hour surveillance, and still refused to talk to us.

The next day Howie and I went alone to visiting hours where we were able to meet with a doctor. By this time Molly had been stabilized and medicated enough that she was willing to see us, but only with a doctor present.

We were like animals in a lab. Our every move, comment, and interaction evaluated against an undisclosed set of criteria. She was the patient, and for some reason we were treated like suspects in an unknown crime.

The only good thing that came out of Dryden was that we finally heard a diagnosis that seemed to fit.

"Given the symptoms Molly is currently exhibiting, and the history we've gathered, we believe we are seeing a clear case of Borderline Personality Disorder."

The first time I heard the words "borderline personality disorder," outside of a textbook during Abnormal Psych in college, was when I read the psych assessment for Molly's birth parents. A psychologist met with them once and wrote, among other things, *Signs of borderline present in both...*

A red flag? Maybe. But what were we to do? It was buried in a much longer document describing their lifestyle as both a cause and effect for much of their instability. I reasoned our child would be raised in an environment vastly different than the one she was born into. I believed with all my heart that any issues she might inherit we could overcome. The classic nature versus nurture controversy and I was sure we would win.

It wasn't until this moment almost seventeen years later that I heard borderline personality disorder again. I had heard lots of diagnoses up until this point: ADHD, ADD, depression, anxiety, autism, Asperger's, and even bipolar. She had symptoms of each, but nothing fit completely or continuously. Nothing fit her whole personality.

When the doctors first mentioned the diagnosis, Molly was still withdrawn and refusing to speak to us. With our connection broken for the moment, I let my mind drift back to her birth parents and entertain the possibility that we were losing the uphill battle we had been fighting for years. Leo and Emily showed no signs of mental illness. Raised in the same household, it seemed logical whatever this was had a genetic component to it.

The doctors explained why borderline is a diagnosis they are hesitant to give until eighteen years of age. Before then, a child's brain is considered too underdeveloped to make the complete diagnosis, and many of the symptoms could go away with further development.

It still didn't make sense to me. *Wouldn't a diagnosis earlier be helpful?* Back then I just accepted what they said and moved on to next steps. As I talked to the doctors and started my own research, I started to understand more why they were so hesitant. Borderline is a personality disorder. By its very definition it says that the patient's personality works against them. The specific symptoms of borderline are:

- An intense fear of abandonment, even going to extreme measures to avoid real or imagined separation or rejection.
- A pattern of unstable, intense relationships, such as

idealizing someone one moment and then suddenly believing the person doesn't care enough or is cruel.
- Rapid changes in self-identity and self-image that include shifting goals and values and seeing yourself as bad or as if you don't exist at all.
- Periods of stress-related paranoia and loss of contact with reality, lasting from a few minutes to a few hours.
- Impulsive and risky behavior, such as gambling, reckless driving, unsafe sex, spending sprees, binge eating or drug abuse, or sabotaging success by suddenly quitting a good job or ending a positive relationship.
- Suicidal threats or behavior or self-injury, often in response to fear of separation or rejection.
- Wide mood swings lasting from a few hours to a few days, which can include intense happiness, irritability, shame or anxiety.
- Ongoing feelings of emptiness.
- Inappropriate, intense anger, such as frequently losing your temper, being sarcastic or bitter, or having physical fights.

I couldn't believe it. Molly exhibited *every single one* of these symptoms to varying degrees. Then why didn't I feel relief? Because as I read further, and talked to more doctors and therapists, I couldn't get my arms around how I would fix this. Of course, meds could control some of the co-existing conditions like anxiety, depression, even some impulsivity with ADHD meds, but nothing could rewire her whole personality. Then I understood. BPD is a lifelong diagnosis—treatable but not curable. Doctors are careful in giving out what, in some way, is a life sentence.

> *Anything that's human is mentionable, and anything that is mentionable can be more manageable. When we can talk about our feelings, they become less overwhelming, less upsetting, and less scary. The people we trust with that important talk can help us know that we are not alone.*
>
> —FRED ROGERS

PART THREE

The Support System

CHAPTER EIGHT

When I Can't Talk, I Type

While Molly was at Dryden, I turned to my computer each night rather than facing a barrage of questions I didn't have the strength to absorb and answer. It was a good coping mechanism, setting a boundary that gave me some control while simultaneously letting in family and friends who were concerned. These are the actual emails I sent during that time.

```
February 28, 2013
8:34 a.m.
"Hi Everyone,
```
Since some of you know and some of you don't, I'm going to give a full update…This past Monday Molly said again she did not feel safe with herself—it is a very long story and I'm not really up to explaining the whole thing, but she was

very hostile to Howie and me. This made no sense to anyone—her counselor at school, us, or her psychiatrist. Things have been going well before she expressed that she didn't feel safe with herself—she was moving forward with her road test, plans for a culinary school, a theater internship, getting a part in a school play.

However, no matter what anyone did or said she was on a mission. Her mission this time was/still is to not live in our home anymore. I don't know why—I only know my little girl was not speaking but someone with a mental illness was. Please understand, all my friends who like me want to fix her because she is broken, and we love her...mental illness does not make sense to a logical mind. There is no root cause and there is no logical path—it is only a path she will lead with ups and downs, and we are only along for the ride—a very bumpy one. As my brother put it—we've done what we could up to 17 (she'll be 17 next week) but we need help to figure out the future—we're out of tricks.

Since she could not commit to being safe with herself or us in our home she was sent via ambulance late yesterday to a facility in Northern NJ—Dryden. She will remain there in Acute Care for a maximum of one week. During her time there she will be assigned a case manager who will help her and us determine the next steps—home, a residential facility, group home

The rest of us? Crap—it sucks worse than anything I've ever experienced. I am so sad I can barely function—sometimes I'm ok and I thank God for all of you and for the rest of my family. My parents flew up yesterday and were able to come with me while I followed the ambulance and Howie finished operating and then took the twins to their High School orientation. He also took them to our therapist where typically, Emily feels sad and guilty, and Leo feels angry—but they are both talking—they are great kids, and they'll be fine.

Please, please understand if I don't want to talk—it is so hard to go through things over and over again—sometimes I'm up for it—sometimes not…I hope you understand because I need you all very much.

Going out for a run now—I am still committed to training for the marathon and Chairing the 8th Grade Dance—the distractions are healthy I know. I am running to my parents where I will let them take care of me today—I will keep you posted as I know more.

xoxoS

March 3, 2013
4:57 p.m.
Hi Everyone,

I know you've all been calling, emailing, texting—it is just hard to talk sometimes so I apologize for the email, but I find it easier for now.

Howie and I went to visit Molly today and for the first time since she was admitted she seemed less hostile and more sad. Our visit was only an hour and very draining, but the three of us did talk about real things—my only definite conclusion is that we have a long road ahead of us. The best part of the visit is that she let me hug her goodbye. I will go back on Tuesday and will bring Leo and Emily for a visit on Thursday—Molly's 17th birthday. We will be in close contact with her case manager this week as we start to figure out where to go from here.

Here, we are taking one day at a time, trying to take good care of each other.

Thank you so much for all your support, encouraging words, and emails and messages full of love—they mean so much—we read them over and over. I do feel more optimistic now that we will get through this, but overwhelmed when I think of what's ahead—and I go back to thinking one day at a time.

xoxoxoS

Molly was released earlier than we expected to an Intensive Outpatient Program *(IOP)*.

March 7, 2013
5:02 p.m.
Hi Everyone,
I want to thank all of you for your calls, emails, deliveries, gifts, and even those special few who were able to join us for lunch today—it made Molly's birthday very special for her. It reminded her how many people care about her—and it helped me make this birthday celebratory—something I did not think I would be able to do. So thank you again—you all made a real difference.

Today has been a good day all around. We found out this morning that Molly will begin her outpatient program tomorrow. She will be picked up by a bus each morning and spend all day in intensive therapy, groups, etc....as well as have school instruction. This will last anywhere from 2-3 weeks and then, hopefully, she will be able to return to school and be bused back to this facility after school several days a week for therapy, etc.… With a lot of hard work from her and all of us, we are hopeful we are on the right path—but we know now that there will probably be some more bumps ahead.

Leo and Emily also had a good day—Leo got his "fisheye lens" for his camera—a gift for getting into Communications High School, and Emily found out she placed into the 2 honors classes she had to take tests for—for the moment all are happy—so…so is mom. Howie will be home tonight and I'm looking forward both to Molly being at a safe, productive place tomorrow—one that is not my living room, as well as sharing some of this with Howie again!!

I love you all—
xoxoS

March 13, 2013
11:38 a.m.
Good Morning,
Thank you again, and over and over again, for all of your calls, support and just being there—whether we are able to talk to you in person or just a quick text it all means so much. What I'm struggling with is that every day has so many ups and downs that when I'm feeling good and able

to talk it's hard to reach out because I know re-hashing what is going on will make me upset again. When things are tough—talking is impossible. So—please continue to understand, and if I've seemed to "avoid" a phone call—I'm sorry— I promise it is not forever and you all mean so very much to our whole family.

That being said—things are progressing. Molly began her day program and the program routine is good. Each day is a challenge and is not without setbacks. There are still a lot of unknowns, and I don't know what her future has in store for her—but for now she is getting the help she needs. She is really trying at home much of the time. Some of the adjustments like be unable to leave her alone or having to lock up the knives, are difficult to accept but we just keep reminding ourselves it is temporary. There are many late-night discussions, lots of tough topics, and walking on eggshells. Family therapy begins this week—I'm happy because I am not a trained therapist and am way too involved and stripped of most of my own coping skills right now to do it all.

Today is sunny—that helps. A good morning run with Pam and I'm meeting Fredda for lunch—last minute and glad to get out. Trying to keep the rest of the house running and holding on by a thread…but I know that will all still be there in a month.

We love you all -
xoxoS

March 29, 2013

12:31 p.m.

Hi Everyone,

Thanks for all of your calls, emails, and texts. And thank you for really understanding our need to cope with this crisis our way—it is so moving when someone just calls/emails…to let us know they are thinking of us with no responsibility left on us…it's like a virtual hug!!

Overall, things are quieted down—I'm just very cautious to say, "for now." Molly began the second phase of her program today, where she goes from 12-5:30 each day. If she continues to do well, she could go back to her school in a little over a week. Once back, she will be picked up there at around 2 each day and go to her program until 5:30—the school portion just moves back to her regular high school.

Things are better—most days now. Molly is working hard and it shows, and we are all working through things in family therapy. The challenge is and will be when she leaves this safe, structured environment and is hit with the real world, everyday challenges. How will she cope? How will we all?

I've learned a new word for me—compartmentalizing. It is not easy for me at all. Howie is much better at it. I'm trying to remember that so much of my life is still good—and I have so many good things in it. Molly's challenges will continue to affect her and all of us. Sometimes more than others. Hopefully, we continue to learn to let that be part of our life—not all of what we're about.

I will continue to update you from time to time—but I do think we are through the major part of this crisis—things could change tomorrow—but today is sunny, we had two beautiful nights of Passover with our family, and Spring Break is finally here!! Today we are all smiling and looking forward to tomorrow—I hope you all are too!!

Much, much love,

Stacy and Howie

What a difference a month makes.

CHAPTER NINE

Therapy. Therapy. And More Therapy.

I am a strong proponent of therapy and am yet to meet anyone who wouldn't benefit from having a professional to talk to now and then. Over the years therapy has been a lifesaver for my family many times over. A place to safely work through current issues. A chance for personal reflection and deeper compassion for one another in a non-judgmental, safe, and when needed—moderated space. To many, Molly seemed the catalyst, although years earlier, when she was still a dream, therapy helped Howie and I get through our struggles with fertility.

Then there was Carl O'Connor.

Dr. O'Connor began as Molly's therapist and eventually saw the whole family individually and in small groups as needed. He was a very kind and soft-spoken man in Bryn Mawr,

Pennsylvania, and our primary therapist for almost five years. We trusted him so much that Molly went back to him for the year she was at college at Temple University.

I don't remember how exactly I found Dr. O'Connor, but I do remember the first time Howie and I went to meet with him. We sat in his office waiting room in the child-sized chairs. Howie, whether to distract himself or me, or both, reached over and picked up one of the sorting toys and began to match the pieces with the correctly shaped holes, both of us fully absorbed in his progress. I sat on my chair holding a growing folder marked *Molly* on my lap. My feet tapped uncontrollably to a beat I didn't hear. When Howie completed the puzzle, I busied myself watching the folder rise and fall. There on top of all the papers lay a list of questions.

Howie and I discussed finding a therapist for Molly. To me it was a natural progression to make her better. Howie was willing to go along with whatever I said. But he didn't drive anything. He seemed much less concerned about her than I was. Maybe it was because he got to leave the house each day to go to work and his job kept him late many nights. He was a colon and rectal surgeon at the University of Pennsylvania and pretty junior in the hierarchy. The work was demanding, the hours were long, and his boss was an ass. I understood how difficult his days were, but I couldn't help feeling jealous. I think it let him stay removed and gave him some perspective. I, on the other hand, was stuck in the weeds every single day and often felt like a hamster on a wheel right back where I started at the end of each day. For every one of my worries, he had a counter. A rosier, glass half-full version. On one hand it kept me balanced. On the other, it made me feel like I was alone on an island screaming for help.

Dr. O'Connor came into the waiting room. An average size, average build, all around average looking guy. But once we sat in his office facing him on the couch as a couple, amidst toys obviously used with many of his patients, I understood why he was recommended.

He listened. Intently. He sat across from us, his legs crossed, looking at us without judgment. Nodding every so often, encouraging us to continue. We talked about Molly's history, the adoption, her performance at school, issues at home, and generally brought him up to speed. The same speech I had been giving to all the specialists and doctors I had been making the rounds to concerning Molly. But he didn't let us stop there. He asked questions that probed and drilled down to our real worries. In that hour when we were supposed to be talking about Molly, we talked about our fears too.

What does this all mean? For her? For now? For her future?

I didn't say it all out loud but knew he heard me loud and clear. At the end of our first hour Dr. O'Connor uncrossed his legs and leaned in. I expected him to give his professional opinion on Molly. Instead, he said, "Molly is going to be fine. I'll meet with her, and we'll work together."

Then he looked directly at me. "It's you I'm worried about. Are you seeing someone?"

I sat back in the couch a little embarrassed. I knew that while I didn't always feel it, I usually gave off an air of control, of having it all together. He was the first person that saw through me—and so quickly.

"Me? Well, we did see someone in New York when we were going through infertility treatment, but now I'm just focused on Molly…"

"I think it would be good for you, and for the whole family if you had someone to talk to."

I liked this man.

"Can you see me too?"

I'm not sure why he was able to see me as Molly was his

client. But for the next couple of years Dr. O'Connor saw Molly regularly, me regularly, occasionally Howie and me as a couple, and even met Leo and Emily. He was always steady and calming and helped us work through many issues that were to come.

When we moved to New Jersey, we were forced to leave Dr. O'Connor. Finding a good therapist means different things to different people. And within everyone's personal criteria are their own changing needs. We bounced around looking for the right fit until we found Dr. Ellman, who as you may recall was referred to us by Dr. Franklin after Molly's first visit to Riverview. A kind, calm, older man—we knew he had a brain tumor when we met him and sadly, he passed away at the end of Molly's junior year in high school. He was instrumental in getting her placed at Windward High School and he helped us understand the changing world of sexual orientation when Molly told us she was a lesbian while at Harmony Teen Camp the summer after freshman year of high school.

Harmony Teen Camp, part of a larger institute where I had attended several yoga retreats over the years, promised "an exciting four-week summer camp for teenagers ages 13–18 years old. This camp is designed to help teenagers find a more peaceful, joyful and positive way to live in the world."

I was sold. It sounded like the perfect antidote to the chaotic and crisis-driven life we had been living all year. A place that could give her tools to manage a personality that was becoming more and more out of balance. I even allowed myself to fast forward, to fantasize what success could look like. She could find her place. A lifestyle, and community, and maybe even a career where she'd be happy, peaceful and productive. I imagined her coming home with a yoga practice all her own, the two of us going to classes together. Maybe she'd even get her certification and teach. I was giddy with the thought and wondered why I hadn't thought of it sooner.

Molly was an easy sell. She was drawn into yoga not so much by the physical practice but the aura surrounding it. Meditation, chanting, candles, incense, it was a mystical world she was more than happy to go play in for four weeks.

I was still congratulating myself three weeks later when I looked at my phone and saw Molly was calling. She was breathless, barely suppressing her excitement, but waited for both of us to be on the phone before she blurted out, "Mom and Dad, I just realized I'm a lesbian!"

We were silent. Now I must take some time here to explain our reaction. I consider both Howie and I liberal and accepting parents, and even in the time period this took place, circa 2009–2010, we would have supported this announcement from any of our children. But, with Molly everything was served in layers requiring patience in the peeling.

So we listened, using the time to digest.

"The whole camp was in a sweat lodge, *(something like a steam room as I understood)* and it got so hot we took off our clothes. Then we started dancing and, well, I really like this one girl…and now we're girlfriends."

I knew I had to be delicate. I tried to sort out the thoughts running through my head.

Oh no, here we go again.

If this is real, no big deal.

How can this be real—her room is plastered with posters of Justin Bieber and Taylor Lautner?

Maybe a freak storm will take out the cell tower and I can deal with this later.

I passed judgment at my own doubts, then remembered this is Molly. I had reason to doubt. She was like a chameleon changing colors to fit her background. But she was Orwellian in her approach, and true to form I heard her insisting she had *always* been a lesbian, even going so far as to accuse us of missing the signs along the way.

"You *know* I've always been more interested in Hermione than Harry."

The call was short, leaving us breathless and thankful for the time to process and prepare before camp ended next week. I wanted my next steps to be the right ones and felt completely out of my league.

I called Dr. Ellman for advice and as always, he delivered.

"While I am not surprised, as Molly looks for ways to both stand out and fit in, I do not believe her to be a lesbian. Her first reaction, whenever we are talking, shows a tendency towards heterosexual interest. However, *(and this was the interesting part)* sexuality is now believed to be on a continuum not an either/or as we used to believe, so she could still be interested in boys and now girls as well."

While this announcement never made social media headlines, it marked a turning point in our lives. Molly continued to explore sexual trends that were new to us but became mainstream to the younger crowd. No longer simply homosexual or heterosexual, gay or straight. Suddenly words like polyamorous, pansexual, demisexual, were thrown at us like tests we continually failed, firmly placing us in the "oh so boring" and "what do we know" *cisgender* category.

The world changed around us. Sexuality, gender, and pronoun terms multiplying faster than I could keep up. I was humble in my ignorance and willing to learn, and in some ways Molly and I connected over her emerging independence. We spoke for hours in hushed voices, both of us trying to be patient. Nothing was out of bounds, and I was grateful she felt accepted in the LGBTQ+ community.

The terms were daunting, and for the first time I could

understand what my parents felt like trying to use the internet or text message. Later that summer I found myself sitting in a big circle with my friends at the beach sharing the many terms that were new to us, commiserating in our own naivete, and wondering when our choices became so out of date, so bland, so vanilla with chocolate sprinkles which just so happens to be my favorite choice of ice cream cone as well.

Dr. Ellman was unable to see me as a patient but referred me to Dr. Sanders.

Dr. Sanders shared an office space with Dr. Ellman, and that is where their similarities ended. Where Dr. Ellman was soft spoken and seemed to process all I said before responding, Dr. Sanders was in your face, part of the conversation, forcing me to look at my situation with a brutal honesty I hadn't yet encountered.

Our first few sessions flew as I filled him in on Molly and the whole family. He got Molly and got her in a way that no one else had to date. He also understood the school system and their ability or lack thereof to support her. He didn't try to repaint the picture I drew, instead encouraging me to *tell it like it is* even when it wasn't pretty.

One day I told him I felt badly about my differences in relationships with Leo and Emily, and Molly. How I worked to keep things fair, but it wasn't always easy because Molly had to be disciplined more. As he got to know all of them through my stories, he summed it up one day in a neat little package that I've held on to since.

"Stacy, why did you have children?"

I just stared at him, not sure where he was going with this.

"I mean it. Why did you have children?"

"Because I always wanted a family. It was all I ever really wanted. Why? I'm not sure what you mean..." I answered with what I thought was honesty.

"Well, let me tell you what I mean. We have children, yes because they're cute, and yes because we want a family. But why do we want that family? It's because we get something from it. Something positive. Some joy. Now, Leo and Emily, while I'm sure they have their moments and it's hectic and tiring and all, they bring you joy. You get something in return. With Molly, though, it's different. There is nothing in return. It's very much a one-way relationship right now."

I had never heard someone lay it out so brutally. It tore through the selfless mommy facade of doing it all and expecting nothing in return. Getting something out of it seemed downright selfish with a red-letter S. But he was right. Being with Molly was all consuming, draining, depleting. I never knew what would happen next, and I lived in fear wondering what it would be.

I paused, drawing from my darkest depths. I tried to take a deep breath before I continued and leaned in close, sharing a secret with this stranger that up until that moment, I'd barely told myself.

"I feel so guilty all the time. Sometimes I'm so angry at her that I want to hurt her feelings, and I don't even care if I leave her crying. And sometimes…I even want to really hurt her."

I inhaled sharply, like I surprised even myself and was trying to take it back. But the words were out there, and they hung between us as I reached for a tissue. I wiped my cheeks, my true feelings pouring out almost as quickly as my tears. The feelings of failure as a mom who feels like, try as I might, things are slipping away. The frustration and anger that come with dealing with Molly and many of the same things since she was a baby, simply in a teenage package, day after day. The guilt for rejecting her when I just can't take it anymore. And finally, the fear that this will never end, that she'll live with us forever, or worse, that it will only end with her ending her life.

He didn't stop me or tell me it was going to be okay, and I respected him for that. I had plenty of friends and family who listened and tried to tell me that. I knew better. I needed Dr. Sanders' honesty. It was a dose of reality in a world that I felt wanted me to keep working toward a fantasy I may never achieve.

"Stacy, all your worries are real and justified. She will always have these problems, but your relationship and how you deal with her will continue to change over the years. But you can stop worrying about one thing today. She doesn't feel things in the same way. So, after you fight when you worry for hours and go to sleep upset—realize she is on to something else. It would take years of rejection for her to feel it and you care too much to let that happen. So, rest easy about that part and we'll work on the rest."

Dr. Sanders also educated me on the disease we were dealing with. Periodically Molly favored one parent over the other. Sometimes it seemed triggered by an event, and other times it was difficult to pinpoint what started it. Recently, there seemed to be an impenetrable wall between Howie and Molly. A far cry from the days she ran to him when he got home from work, these days she wouldn't talk to or even look at him. She began referring to him in the third person. As a result, I became the sole object of Molly's affection. Her go to for all things from hour-long soliloquies on any topic she chose to problems at school.

"I feel so alone. It's like I've become both mom and dad when it comes to Molly. I try to step in, reprimand her when she refuses to pass Howie something at the table or calls him *your husband*. But I just can't seem to fix this, and Howie says he's not going to change her mind, so he just ignores her."

Dr. Sanders smiled knowingly. "Well, Howard is right. You're not going to fix it. Molly is splitting."

"Splitting?" I asked.

"Yes. Splitting is very common in people with borderline. It's when they view the world in extremes, as all good or all bad. Right now, you are all good and Howie all bad. It will probably continue until either she stops getting what she wants out of it this way, or you do something that makes her angry enough to see you as all bad. I know it's frustrating, but relax, these perceptions also tend to change quickly."

Dr. Sanders' office became a safe place where I shed any pretenses. I dug deep, uncovering feelings I didn't even know I had or was too ashamed to admit to anyone else, even myself. He helped me take off any rose-colored glasses I wore and face the reality of a worsening situation.

Dr. Sanders never actually met Molly, but I marveled at how spot on he was about her and stopping me when I edited stories, reminding me to say what I really feel not what I thought I should say or feel. I needed to be past that. At least with myself. At least in his office.

And last, but definitely not least, to complete our therapist support system was Marnie Gellman. Marnie began as our in-home therapist after Molly was at Dryden. She was assigned by the Monmouth County services to help the whole family cope with Molly's illness. I didn't know what to expect but it was easy, and it was free, and I was willing to try anything.

I made sure everyone was home and promised them we just had to try. Family counseling was new to us, and I didn't know what to expect. Up until this point I had played family counselor and mediator, and I was tired and out of tricks. Keeping the peace while making sure everyone was heard and valued often felt like an Olympic event. Sometimes I wondered if closing my eyes, covering my ears, and screaming until my throat was raw would work better. I never tried.

Since Molly got home from Dryden and began her Intensive

Outpatient Program *(IOP)*, we were all on our best behavior. It was always like this. She wore us down with erratic and explosive, almost abusive behavior until a crisis. Then the honeymoon period—when she was taking her treatment seriously, even taking her meds. This time she said she was relieved to finally have a diagnosis, something to explain her to her. She was processing it all and piecing it together in her own way. I hoped it would help her understand but not become an excuse. I just wanted her to keep moving forward. She was in her junior year, and it was time to start thinking about post-grad plans. Dr. Ellman broached the possibility of a fifth year of high school. I listened politely with no intention of pursuing that avenue. Instead, I focused on a newfound energy, even, dare I say hope? I was in touch with her school, coordinating transportation between her IOP and Windward, assuring her work is done in both places, and trying to keep any progress made inside the hospital and the IOP continuing on the outside.

The others? I think they were just glad for the peace. Leo and Emily were busy with their social lives, as fourteen-year-olds should be, and seemingly thankful for no more emotional interruptions. At a time when they want to blend in, an unexpected trip to a mental hospital is hard to coolly explain away to their friends. Howie was busy with work, not uninvolved, but much better able to separate than me.

Marnie Gellman became part of our family from the moment she first walked in the front door. Her easy, bright smile looking up at me when I opened the door immediately put me at ease. Her long, dark curls held back by a single clip on top of her head made her look like any friend who might stop by, and her casual yet direct nature drew us all in as we found our places around the living room.

Marnie fell comfortably into one end of our L-shaped

couch as if she were an old friend coming for a visit. She tucked one leg under another, dropped her binder and notes next to her, and looked around the room almost excitedly as if to say, "Okay let's get this meeting started!"

The rest of us were polite at first, scattered around the remaining seating. Molly sat next to Marnie in the corner of the L, her feet sticking straight out. Emily rested her head on my chest on the far end of the couch, and Howie and Leo found seats in the blue club chairs rounding out our circle.

Over the course of the next hour Marnie drew us out, asking each of us what was going on. She began with her actual client, Molly, and I could tell immediately underneath her relaxed demeanor was a no-nonsense professional who seemed to really understand Molly. It was almost as if she knew her. Like she knew our family—or at least what we were going through.

She called Molly out when she was using her diagnosis as an excuse and dug deeper with Leo and Emily than anyone else about how hard it must be for them. I cried silently when Emily talked about how she felt scared Molly was going to kill herself and how angry she was when Molly stole from her. I listened quietly as Leo opened up about how he hates what Molly is doing to our family and just can't understand why she does it. I even let Howie talk for the short time he did about the good times, how well Molly was doing now, and how he just wanted everyone to be okay. I choked on my words as I filled in the details and described some of our nighttime or dinner experiences ending in yelling, slammed doors, or worse.

Marnie was both a facilitator and a referee, ensuring everyone had their time to speak without interruptions. Her presence kept our discussions from heating up past our boiling point. She seemed an ally to all of us, genuinely interested in our family.

Over the course of our time working with her, Marnie

became an ally, and at some point, we became friends. I used our visits as a place to work through things that happened between sessions. Early on we were all there regularly, but as time went on Molly, Emily, and I were the most consistent attendees. On more than one occasion, Marnie stopped Molly from storming out, forcing us to work completely through something and seeing the effects of her actions.

Marnie had a special affinity for Emily and for Leo, as siblings, and through her I learned how deeply they were affected by Molly's illness. It was painful to hear, but with Marnie's guidance I listened and was able to face the revision to the fairytale childhood I had planned. Slowly I accepted their sadness, fear, frustration, and anger for what it was—normal given the circumstances. And I started to believe what Dr. O'Connor, Dr. Ellman, Dr. Sanders, and Marnie had been telling me—none of it was my fault or my personal failure. Maybe our family life wasn't the fairytale I had dreamed of, but for the first time, I entertained the idea that our fairytale could still be rewritten.

―― CHAPTER TEN ――

It's Not Easy Being Married to Superman

Molly's mental illness was beyond anything we thought we understood. When she was first diagnosed with borderline personality disorder, I reacted in the only way I knew how. I doubled down and worked harder. As BPD cannot be fixed in the way I hoped back then, all I had were treatments to alleviate the symptoms and help make her the best version of herself.

Dialectical behavioral therapy *(DBT)*, created by Dr. Marsha Linehan, was considered to be the best way to treat BPD at the time. DBT is a type of talk therapy. According to the Cleveland Clinic, "DBT focuses on helping people accept the reality of their lives and their behaviors as well as helping them learn to change their lives, including their unhelpful behaviors."

Unfortunately, Molly was reluctant and ultimately refused to even try DBT therapy. So I, the fixer, was faced with a mental illness that could not be fixed and a child who refused to try the treatment that was proven to help. It both saddened and infuriated me.

By the end of high school, we were living crisis to crisis. Every day was surreal—it didn't make sense, and I never knew what would happen next. Only in hindsight do I realize this is when I started developing a coat of armor in an attempt to deflect the almost daily onslaught.

For much of this time, my toolbox of coping skills gathered dust. Instead, I ran on the adrenalin of constantly trying to stay one step ahead.

I attached myself to Molly as best as I could. Instead of strategically choosing which battles to fight, I chose every single one. I stopped letting anything slide.

I woke her up every morning, cutting off her protests and complaints with a command.

"You have a half hour until the bus comes and you will be on it."

I went back in every two minutes, and if she wasn't showing signs of moving, I picked out her clothes and put her into a sitting position myself, chiding her into an immediate confrontation.

"You don't have to do that, *Mother, I am up!*"

Not a pleasant way to start the day but it did the trick.

Afternoons weren't much different. I watched the clock, my heart sinking and my anxiety climbing a bit as the minutes passed. When I heard her bus pull away and the garage door go up, I squared my shoulders and met her at the back door with the same greeting every day.

"Hi, sweetie. How was your day? What homework do you have?"

I held my breath hoping for the best.

I usually got a grunt, followed by a promise to get to her homework right after a "quick nap." I rarely stopped her, instead welcoming a little more peace. It gave me time to spend with Leo and Emily, help them with homework, and get dinner ready. While she slept, our household felt normal and I relished it, blasting ABBA as I cooked.

I knew I had to wake her to get the work done. Or I would be right back in the middle of a barrage of emails that continued to chip away at me every day.

I climbed the steps as slowly as I could and started all over again. Most nights either my throat was raw from yelling and the work was done, or I let her sleep, we had a peaceful dinner, and she went to school empty handed.

No matter what I did, it seemed I lost.

Was I supposed to learn something from all of this? In retrospect, I was always searching for ways to recreate the fairytale. But maybe the search is what created the stand-off. Molly's behavior, that I often called childlike with a negative connotation, also carried with it the wonderment of childhood. Molly's traits, many of the symptoms of borderline and all its co-existing conditions, also have beauty in them. Let me explain.

Molly is uninhibited, impulsive, and unable to understand situational expectations—in other words she cannot *read a room*. I believed it my job to help her manage these symptoms so she could fit in and be an accepted part of society. Maybe fitting in is overrated. With the exception of my college years *(and even then, I wasn't completely uninhibited)*, I cannot recall a time my brain didn't have some sort of mental checklist of how I should be acting, what I should be saying, or how I was affecting others. I performed well, but sometimes performing is exhausting.

Molly just *was*.

I never let her out of my sight at family events. I remember the bat mitzvah of the daughter of my college roommate. I watched her enter a circle of our closest family friends. It both broke my heart and drove me crazy in anticipation of what was coming. She didn't seem to worry at all.

The conversation already flowing, Molly stepped in and laughed at the last comment too loudly, stopping the chatter dead in its tracks. All eyes turned to her, tolerant smiles spreading across their faces. I quickly joined and opened my mouth trying to restart the easy flow. Before I got a word out, Molly filled the silence, her pre-teen voice high pitched and sped up like an Instagram or TikTok influencer.

"Have you heard the latest Justin Bieber song? I know all the words. He's so cute. I just love his hair. I've been asking my mom to go to the concert. Do you want me to sing it for you? I hope the band plays some Justin Bieber songs…"

On and on, trapping us in a circular soliloquy, all adults too polite to interrupt. I didn't miss the eye rolling though luckily, she did. I reached out and gently touched her arm hoping to signal or break her train of thought.

She swatted me away, recoiling as if I burned her. "What, Mom? Why are you touching me?"

All eyes on me now, calling more attention to what already felt like a hostage situation.

Gail, my college roommate, tried to lighten the mood.

"Wow, Molly, you know a lot about Justin Bieber. He is very cute!" Her comment released the tension enough to give everyone a polite way out. One by one the rest of the group stepped away.

The rest of the night passed without incident, and I resisted the urge to apologize. Later that night when she was getting ready for bed, I went into her room and brought it up.

"Molly, when you were talking about Justin Bieber today, you didn't give anyone else a chance to speak."

"I know everything about him, Mom, and I just love him. No one cared."

"Yes, they did, they were just too polite to interrupt you. When you step into a group you need to listen before you speak. And when you're talking, try to give everyone else a chance…"

"Well, if they have something to say they should just speak up!" she insisted.

I sighed.

Enter social skills training classes, behavioral charts, signals for when we were out, and reviewing social interactions at bedtime each night. But it wasn't and still isn't lost on me that being Molly also means holding on to that freedom of expression that most of us lose, or at least carefully manage by the time we are teenagers. Fitting in becomes much more important.

But without the social constraints the rest of us become shackled with, Molly's reactions were impulsive, yes, but beautifully uncurated—as honest and real as a child opening a present and screaming with glee.

So while I may have cringed when she sang the loudest at temple or danced alone on a dance floor or did a cartwheel where a polite thank you would have been more appropriate, it was only Molly being herself, more truly herself than many of us ever are.

True Molly Fashion.

We called it True Molly Fashion, and in the confines of our own home, with no one else around to judge or to worry about, we were able to breathe a little easier and enjoy some of her *moments*. In fact, her impulsivity combined with her intelligence made for some of our funniest stories. One time we were having a whole group of surgery residents over for Rosh Hashanah dinner. I invited anyone over who was too far from family to go home. No one should be alone for a holiday.

It seemed like a good idea at the moment, but in the thick of the usual afternoon chaos, while preparing dinner for twenty, I wondered what I was thinking.

I was moving at high speed in the kitchen, barking orders through to the living room at the kids like a drill sergeant.

"Put away your toys."

"Turn off the TV."

"Emily, you're dancing again, do you have to go to the bathroom?"

"Leo, please go upstairs and put on the shirt I put out for you?"

"Molly…Molly…"

No answer.

She's too quiet. Where is she?

I took off the oven mitts and strode across the kitchen, poised to pounce and get back to preparing dinner as quickly as possible.

I stepped into the TV room and stopped dead in my tracks. There she was, sitting quietly on our leather recliner, her eyes covered with cucumbers she had taken from the vegetable platter already out for our guests.

"I'm meditating, Mom, so I'm ready for our guests."

It was a great tension release. I laughed until the tears came.

Oh, how I longed to lighten up and laugh like that more often, but this all was so heavy. I wondered if Dr. O'Connor was right being worried about me as I worried so much about Molly.

Howie's approach was so different, which sometimes drove me just as crazy. He never seemed as worried as me. When the kids were little, he was out of the house a lot, a young surgeon building his practice and his reputation. I stopped working to take care of the kids full time. It was my dream, but the reality was very different. It always felt like it was all on me. Howie was willing to do whatever I asked, but sometimes I wanted him to drive the boat, not just come along for the ride.

As the rollercoaster of Molly's crises built speed, we made room for each other to cope in our own ways and then figure out how we would face them together. Since I was with Molly most, I knew how to manage her best. When Howie got home, he jumped in where he thought he was most helpful, which usually ended up being with the twins. More often than not, I found myself listening to giggles coming from the other rooms, while I was trapped in homework hell in Molly's room.

While I knew he meant well, and would do whatever I asked, I resented Howie getting those fun times with the twins while I was stuck policing Molly's every move, only relaxing when she was finally asleep for the night. When all was finally quiet, Howie reached for me, but I often felt like those arms were asking for more than I had left to give.

As the years wore on and Molly's BPD took over our house, we stayed dedicated to each other, first and foremost. We took those date nights, we celebrated anytime we could, and we laughed—a lot. Don't get me wrong, we also argued, even all out fought, and many of those were purely taking out our frustrations on the one person who would take it. Howie is much more even tempered than I am. He says he loves my passion, but like anything, sometimes it's the things you fall in love with that come back to bite you.

While we lived in Philadelphia, Howie started dressing up like Superman on the first day of school every year and appearing at the neighborhood bus stop to wish the kids a good year. While in costume, Howie carried himself like a superhero, puffing out his chest, deepening his voice, and standing at attention with his legs wide and hands on his hips. He looked every bit the part—so much so I began to wonder if he believed it! It was a fun and playful start to every school year, helping alleviate any first day jitters. Superman continued to make appearances at all family events throughout their childhood and wished them good luck every school year even appearing at their cars when the bus stop was a distant memory.

In many ways Howie really is Superman. He loves stepping in to save the day. When things get tough, he stays maddeningly calm. Instead of being comforting, this often made me feel like he was detached, or didn't understand the gravity of the situation, or just assumed I would handle it. Or worse, it made me feel like I was a failure, unable to handle what he so easily could.

When Molly was admitted to Dryden Clinic and we first heard the diagnosis of BPD, it wasn't the first time she was an in-patient, but it was the first time I felt like she had something that was out of my league. I didn't know how to cope and yet I had to wake up every morning and take care of the kids, the house, and run a yoga studio.

I asked Dr. Sanders how I was supposed to handle this. Not just that first day, but all the days that followed. It was what he said that really made me understand my husband.

In his signature no-nonsense approach, he made it seem doable, even simple. "You will compartmentalize, Stacy. This is just one part of your life. You will learn."

I realized then that Howie wasn't detached, or uncaring, or pushing off the burden, he was compartmentalizing. It was how he was able to reach for me at night after a knock down drag out fight with Molly just minutes earlier. It was how he was able to enjoy our dates after the chaos we left behind. And it was how he was able to focus on his patients and operate no matter what else was going on in his life.

I looked at Howie differently after this. I started to learn from him. With the resentment at bay, I was able to tell him calmly, the way he likes to hear things, what I needed from him. He started to understand that I needed him to take over sometimes purely to give me a break, even if it wasn't the most efficient way of dividing and conquering. I needed the giggling. I craved the lightness. In order get there, I didn't need a different life. I just needed the chance to loosen my grip on this one sometimes.

But loosening my grip was hard. No matter how many breaks I took, or how much help Howie was giving me, I was in an ongoing conflict with Molly that continued to escalate more and more. She became confrontational and combative. I was constantly torn between enjoying the peace when she wasn't home—and feeling guilty about it—to wanting her close by at all times.

So much yelling. So much fighting, So much conflict.

I couldn't fix anything.

The shoes kept falling.

Faster and faster.

Back and forth.

Up and down.

A phone call from the police telling us they brought her to the hospital after she became violent at home.

A phone call from Molly crying to please come pick her up—things would be different.

A phone call from the hospital a few hours later telling us they couldn't keep her—and offering no suggestions on what to do next.

A phone call from Molly telling us she'd been arrested.

Life itself is the most wonderful fairy tale.

-HANS CHRISTIAN ANDERSON

PART FOUR

Lost and Found

—— CHAPTER ELEVEN ——

A Picture Is Worth a Thousand Words and a Transfer

"This is my daughter. I haven't seen her in a while. I'd like you to help us find her again," Howie said, holding up an adorable picture of Molly looking happy and carefree, his voice cracking under the weight of his plea.

There wasn't a dry eye in the conference room.

Molly wasn't really lost in the true sense of the word, but Howie wasn't lying either. By tenth grade the bullying at our public high school had become so unbearable that we couldn't remember the last time we saw her looking happy. Dr. Ellman suggested we ask for district funding to send her to Windward High School. Windward was an alternative high school designed for children with diagnoses that made them outcasts at their public high school. Approval for her transfer depended on us demonstrating they could no longer keep her safe.

We understood we had one chance to prove our case, and we came prepared. Howie, usually dressed in scrubs or at the most jeans and a sports jacket, put on a full suit and a tie. I swapped my yoga clothes for black pants and a blouse. We didn't usually play up our degree-packed resumes, but when it came to advocating for our daughter, we were determined to do what we could to level the playing field.

We walked up the steps to the front doors of the high school, holding hands. We were welcomed by a student greeter and a security guard who checked our name off a list and directed us to a conference room on the second floor. The team was already seated when we walked in.

I knew most of the faces at the table and was glad to see such a large group. While this meeting coincided with our usual Individualized Education Plan *(IEP)* update, it was obvious by the additional attendees they were taking our concerns seriously.

The head of the child study team stood up as we walked in.

"Good morning, Dr. and Mrs. Ross. After speaking to you, I asked some of Molly's teachers and our principal to join us."

She made the necessary introductions, and we sat down at the two open seats in the middle of the long table. I put my pocketbook on the floor next to me and took out my binder, marked Molly in black sharpie down the spine, thick from years of IEP evaluations, reports, doctors visit notes, and any other evaluations or articles I kept on hand. I opened it to a blank page of lined paper. Ready to go.

I took a deep breath and looked around trying to read the

faces at the table. Some had their heads over open notebooks; others met my gaze with a smile. Overall, the room felt welcoming.

As we waited for someone to start the meeting I reached under the table and put my hand on Howie's knee. His hand covered mine, stopping it from shaking. Suddenly a loud bell rang, signaling the start of the next class period. There were no students present, and we weren't waiting for anyone else, so it seemed funny that that was what we were waiting for. But it was. I almost laughed out loud when, in unison, the educators and staff around us sat at attention when the bell rang. The meeting began as soon as it was quiet again.

We let the business of a usual IEP meeting take place around us. It was a reporting of Molly's status in all her classes. The updates were nothing new. Unlike in elementary and middle school where the teachers were somehow able to look past her late homework and find her potential, high school teachers saw only her shortfalls.

"Her homework is always late, and if I see it, it is illegible."

"She can be very disruptive."

"Even with my reminders she doesn't do the work that is assigned."

Molly had plenty of accommodations, each designed to help her focus and give her the most chances for success in school. But they were limited by design. It didn't help that the teachers reminded her of homework or even wrote it down for her unless they were going to come home and make her do it. That was my burden. And then, there was still the question of getting it to class and handing it in. Each step became an opportunity for her to mess up—something she seemed to be doing more and more.

After Howie spoke, our fate was sealed.

We told them some of the bullying stories. Once Molly

started telling us what was going on, it was as if we pulled a cork and the stories kept flowing, each one more disturbing than the last.

One boy locked her out of the school whenever she stepped into the courtyard between buildings, making her late for her next class.

Another boy tried to light her on fire with a Stryker from chem class—the teacher seeming to look the other way.

And that was just the boys.

The girls were less obvious but even meaner—excluding her or worse, engaging her in a way that made her trust them and then embarrassing her in front of a class or a boy that she liked. She was just a toy that they played with and tossed aside when done.

After what we shared, the rest was easy. We all agreed she wasn't safe there anymore. I was prepared to threaten and use the legal rights I had researched as argument, but none of it was needed. Maybe they were as happy to get rid of her as we were to get her out of there. I didn't stop to think about it. We were getting what we wanted. We thanked everyone, gathered our things and left quickly, afraid to look back as if they would realize they just approved a $36,000 line item for the district budget and try to take it back.

As I learned more about Windward, what really stuck out to me was the promise of a safe place for the bullied not the bullies. It was not for children with drug problems or kids on the autism spectrum. There were plenty of schools and support for kids with those challenges. In my initial research, Windward seemed like a school for all the kids who were different enough that they had trouble at their public high school but had the ability and potential to succeed in school. I didn't even mind it was attached to a convent—I'd take any additional support we could get!

Dr. Ellman was one of the psychologists on the Board at Windward and he helped us schedule a tour in record speed. It was that very quiet time between Thanksgiving and Christmas when nothing seemed to get done except shopping and holiday parties. We hoped to speed the process along so that Molly could start there right after the new year. New year, new school. I was feeling very hopeful.

We drove to Windward for the first time on a crisp day in early December. It was about a twenty-minute drive to our house into the horse country of Colts Neck. The roads were windy, and Windward was set on a hill just past a defunct mental health inpatient facility. The irony was not lost on me. As we made our way up the hill, the trees parted and welcomed us to campus. Multiple buildings surrounded a large green open space, making the picturesque setting feel more like a college campus than a school for students with special needs. The buildings themselves were in slight disrepair, highlighting the difference between a private college campus and a school publicly funded by the sending districts of its students.

We were welcomed almost immediately by the principal. Tom Bard was a slick looking man slightly older than Howie and me. He had an easy smile and a casual air about him, putting us all at ease. We sat in the conference room just outside the main office. He knew our story. He had the referral from both Dr. Ellman and Molly's school as well as some preliminary paperwork I had filled out. He spent the time getting to know Molly.

I enjoyed watching them talk. In some ways she seemed so grown up. She had absolutely no problem carrying on a conversation with an adult. In fact, if not for the background, Mr. Bard would probably be wondering why we were here at all.

It was with her own age group that she failed miserably.

So immature that she was dangerously naive with teens. And so socially isolated that she would do almost anything to be part of the group. It was heartbreaking, yet a part of me understood. Molly was not someone who I would have wanted to be friends with when I was in high school. I like to think I wouldn't have made fun of her—I wouldn't have to her face, but behind her back…I'm not so sure.

Gossip is a way of fitting in. Talking about other people builds comradery. There's no getting around that. It isn't until you realize your life, or someone in it, is gossip-worthy that you begin to think twice about participating. There's no excuse for what the kids did to Molly or how I was when I was younger. But Molly did teach me a lot about myself. I realized through the mirror Molly held up for me that I didn't like that part of myself.

Gossip hurts. And whatever you tell yourself to feel better, the people you are gossiping about—*the gossipees*—do know. I never missed the eye rolling or under breath comments of other parents and children. In the local restaurants, at school events, and while volunteering for the PTA and townwide events, I listened and watched. Sometimes it was about other kids in town. On those occasions, when they were talking about him/her for something minor, I only imagined what they were saying about Molly.

Other times it was a little more direct, but still vague. Upon meeting me they barely made eye contact, and said something like:

"Oh, you're Molly's mom…"

"I've heard about Molly from my daughter."

"How's Molly doing? Is she okay?"

Then there were the direct hits.

We were at the middle school for Leo and Emily's talent show. Emily was on stage emceeing the event. I was in the back, standing and taking pictures when Molly walked in with Howie. The lights were already out but my eyes adjusted, and I saw everything.

Molly was wearing a very low-cut shirt with a short, tight skirt and spike-heeled black booties. She was far from the tiny little sixth grader that had entered school here five years earlier. Her hair was dyed blue, with streaks of white after losing a bet on last week's Giants game. It was as if she fell into the room, unaware the lights were out, and a show was in progress.

"Mom?" she said loud enough for Emily to hear on stage.

I waved frantically with one hand while the other came right to my lips.

"Shh..."

It was too late. While I couldn't see anyone rolling their eyes, I could hear the barely veiled whisper of one of my neighbors.

"Can you believe it? Look at that shirt. I can't believe anyone would let their child out in that."

My stomach started burning, my hands itching to slap her, shut her right up. At the very least I wanted her to know I heard her.

As Molly walked back to meet me, I gave her a big hug trying to shield her from the words being spoken. The neighbor's gaze followed Molly, and I stared unblinkingly at that gossip until her eyes landed on me. I threw all my anger into my gaze until her head turned away.

I know I shouldn't have cared. And I still work hard at not caring. But it's hard. I am a mother. I am proud of my children. So, it follows that critique of my mothering hurt. How could it not?

Today when I see a child dancing on a table in a restaurant, talking too loudly, dressed in their own style, even calling their mother names, I don't judge, and I don't talk about the child or the mom. Instead, I smile at them, even offer to help if I can, and do anything to make them feel less isolated than I know they already do.

While Molly continued to speak with Mr. Bard in the small conference room on that cold day in December, her intellect and personality were on full display, and I was reminded of how much she had to offer. I felt something I hadn't felt in a while, certainly not since high school began...hope.

Afterward, we went on a tour around campus. Molly and Mr. Bard walked ahead of Howie and me. She skipped alongside him, talking excitedly about her latest interests, mostly her obsession with Justin Bieber. As she babbled on, I kept quiet, holding back from stopping her like I did so often. Mr. Bard didn't miss a beat, stopping frequently to introduce her to teachers and students alike. He knew everyone, and as we continued our tour I reached for Howie's hand and took my laser gaze off Molly, taking in the setting instead.

The tour ended outside, right next to our car, and Mr. Bard's attention turned to us. His smile looked promising, but I didn't want to misread or leave anything to chance.

"What happens now?"

"Well, since we only have a week left until winter break, it makes the most sense for Molly to begin January 2nd when we return to school."

Smiles broke out all around.

He told me how transportation and paperwork would work and who I needed to get in touch with. Finally, he turned to Molly who was wandering around close by.

"So, Molly, we'd love to have you join our sophomore class. What do you think about that?"

Her answer, in true Molly fashion, was a cartwheel kicking up the dirt from the gravel parking lot.

We all laughed—it was hard not to be caught up in her excitement.

"Wow, that's the best reaction I've ever gotten!"

The next couple of weeks passed easily and quickly. We wrapped things up at NJ Regional. I guessed she was hopeful, because she did what she needed to finish her classes. And for once I didn't worry about her grades.

On a clear morning in early January, a small school bus pulled up to our house and Molly was off to Windward. It was the first time I could remember that she got out of bed without a fight. Her excitement was directly proportional to the relief I felt. As the bus drove away, I felt a lightness I hadn't felt in a long time.

After countless other starts, it was not lost on me that we were once again in the *honeymoon phase*. All her social skills training, and the hours I spent reviewing what was *appropriate* behavior, and maybe even some basic imprinting from being our daughter, seemed to have made an impact and she knew what to do. Without the distractions of bullying, and with the celebrity status that came along with being the new student to a group of children who had all been outcasts, she bounced through the front door every day filled with stories of new friends, teachers who loved her, and a list of activities to get involved in.

Like all honeymoons, this one ended and it wasn't long before the phone started ringing and my inbox filled up again. Same message, different messengers. Molly was not handing in her work, she was a distraction in class, and a new one started to emerge...she wasn't showing up for all her classes. It seemed the open campus style of Windward gave way to more hanging out, and she often *got lost* between classes, many times never making it at all.

Before long, we were right back where we started. I bit my

tongue every afternoon when she got off the bus, just asking about her day. She was usually sullen and sleepy after an hour-long bus ride, and it was easier to let her go up to her room and nap rather than start right in with the burning question that would determine the rest of the evening.

"What do you have for homework?"

Even though it's the mantra of every open school night I've been to—*homework is your child's responsibility, not yours* and *she needs to learn to advocate for herself*—it was still my phone that rang incessantly and my inbox that became flooded when it wasn't getting done.

She ignored me. She told me she didn't feel well. She begged for more sleep. She asked to talk to me about something that happened at school. She had bottomless excuses.

Still, we were surprised when Howie and I went to our first parent night that we were held back by several of the teachers all with similar stories, each one just like what we heard at NJ Regional High School.

"Molly has three, four, five, outstanding assignments."

"I've tried seating her right in front so she can only look at me, but it hasn't helped."

"She seems to have some friends, but many of her classmates get annoyed at her."

I always read between their feedback, wondering what they were really saying. I reminded myself this was a school for children like Molly so why did they seem not to like her, to single her out in a supposedly similar population? I wanted to fix this. I thought Windward was the answer.

After visiting the classrooms, all the parents gathered in the auditorium for a welcome speech from the principal. While Mr. Bard spoke, I looked around at the other parents, wondering what their kid was here for. Unlike similar nights in our home district, I didn't feel like people were pointing at us whispering,

"Those are Molly's parents." Here, there were parents from all walks of life, many coming straight from work wearing everything ranging from suits, to scrubs, to coveralls with fresh grease stains. Some were there alone, and others holding hands with their same sex partners. I did not feel judged at all by these parents, instead I took the time to look around forming my own opinions, making up stories as I went. It's sad I was judging the very people I wanted to accept us. Instead of introducing myself, I stood back with Howie, smiling politely but stopping short of mingling. I believed we were different than the other parents and Windward was simply a detour to help Molly get back on track—the track we laid out. Like an oven, it would cook her till she was ready to be served to the real world.

We saw Mr. Bard on our way out and stopped to say hello. After all the negative feedback I was sure Mr. Bard would right the situation and assure us, late homework assignments aside, how well Molly was doing. He greeted us by name and made small talk asking us about our evening. When I told him about the concerns raised by Molly's teachers, he became serious and turned to face us, cutting off others from joining our small circle.

"I know. I've spoken to her teachers and Molly's in-school therapist *(every student at Windward was assigned an in-school therapist)*. Even in this population, Molly is one of the more severe students we have."

My heart dropped and I took a step back trying put distance between what he just said. Howie looked truly puzzled. I let Mr. Bard's words sink in. So, even in a population where each child has *challenges,* Molly still stands out? I felt the pedestal I had put myself on being pulled out from under me. This was new ground all together. Until this moment I had still been sure she would conquer Windward, graduate top of her class, and easily add to their college acceptance rate. While Mr. Bard's words shocked me, they gave me a glimpse of a reality that I was still only ready to take in small doses.

CHAPTER TWELVE

The Jury Is Out

It's funny how some moments in our lives are really critical shifts in our journey, only viewable in hindsight. Often the instant of change shakes you like an earthquake, recognizing only then the prophetic tremors, a series of conversations, a meeting, or the dreaded phone call.

I had just packed up my things and was leaving the yoga studio. Teaching a weekly yoga class helped me stay connected to the community and the practice without the headaches that came from owning my own studio. The one-hour class created a layer of peace and calm protection from the stressors that flew like a hailstorm during the rest of the week.

I sat down in my car, deciding what I was going to order for lunch at the diner where I was meeting my parents. They came home from Florida earlier in the month, and we had settled comfortably into our summer routine of lunches at the diner, Sunday dinners at my house, and usually one other visit during the week. Still vibrant and active at seventy-six and seventy-seven, there were few things they liked more than spending time with my family, and their relationship with all three of my children and my husband reflected it. Avid golfers and perpetually social, their calendar was often hard to be penned into, although a call from me asking for a lunch date magically erased whatever other plans they had.

Just as I started the car, my phone rang, and while I didn't recognize the number, I picked up. Now I swore I wasn't answering the phone again, but as a mom that's just not an option.

It was Molly.

Molly's years at Windward came with their own challenges. As her BPD symptoms continued to emerge, we found ourselves constantly caught in the crossfire, our home an active battlefield at its worst and a cold war at its best. Molly grew up and grew distant all at the same time. The disease seemed to be taking her over from the inside out and it became harder and harder to find compassion for the stranger she became. Explosive confrontations, violent threats, and constant lies took over most remnants of the little girl Howie was looking for in the conference room at NJR.

My feelings toward Molly were all over the place. Sometimes I applauded her efforts, at other times I welcomed her absence and resented when her chaos blew in the front door. Other times I thought all day long about how to fix things, meeting her head on at the pass with a new plan. Other times I'd approach her tentatively with a measure of empathy, trying to just enjoy some quality time together, hoping for a way in. We had moments of beautiful time together from seeing a Broadway show to a family vacation to Hawk's Cay in Florida. The beginning of that trip was not without trepidation, but as the days wore on, I found myself relaxing into it. We went paddleboarding, laid in the sun, played games, and went on family runs. On our last night there, we held hands and looked up at the night sky. I leaned over and whispered, "You did great."

She leaned down and kissed my hand whispering, "I know.

I love you, Mama." I let the tears run down my cheek, holding on tight to this moment for as long as I could.

Now, with just a few months left until high school graduation, things were looking up and had been for most of the school year. Since going away this past summer to Camp Jumpstart, "a weight loss camp designed for teens who were bullied and didn't fit in at home," she lost weight, was taking better care of herself physically and emotionally, and for the first time she was making plans for the future.

In the fall she announced she wanted to take the SATs and go to Temple University where Howie was working. If accepted, she would have free tuition and a chance to build her future in a place we were familiar with. I tried to balance my hopes, cautiously leaning into this big decision of hers. She applied and was accepted!

She continued to build on that success. She had a lead in *Seussical the Musical*, set to open in a few weeks and was making plans to go to senior prom. While I hadn't seen a report card, my inbox was light on Windward emails. And like high school seniors all over the country she told anyone who would listen about her post-grad plans. It was so quiet—and so normal. And like anyone who has lived from crisis to crisis we embraced it, lulled into a false sense of hope that this was the way it would always be.

So, when the unfamiliar number appeared on the phone and I answered to the sound of Molly's voice, I was reluctantly jolted back to a reality I had hoped we were done with but had never stopped waiting for. I knew it was strange she was calling in the middle of the day. Any phone calls were usually made by her school-assigned therapist, a number I had stored in my contacts. And she had her own phone for personal calls. Pondering on the how of the call was cut short when I was swept up in the absurdity of the why.

"Mom, I fucked up. I was arrested."

Some noise in the background that could have been papers shuffling or just the sound of a phone being passed, and a male voice replaced Molly introducing himself as Sergeant *something or other*. His name was not important, all I could think of was the gravity of the situation that was unfolding. I tried to focus but couldn't hear the details and was instead stuck on the words my oldest child, on the verge of graduation, college acceptance in hand, had just uttered.

"I. Was. Arrested."

I reached into the emotional toolbox that I'd barely used this school year, but how to handle an arrest wasn't something I was prepared for. I broke into a cold sweat, the calm buzz I had earned over the past hour shedding faster than our yellow lab in the summer heat. I took a deep breath and tried to shake my head into focus; I needed to understand what this stranger was saying, what we were up against, and figure out how we were going to deal with it.

In matter-of-fact terms the Sergeant explained Molly had been arrested at her high school after they received a call that another student had overdosed. Apparently, Molly had given the classmate two of her meds that Molly carries with her, with approval from her psychiatrist, as emergency relief from anxiety. He said Molly claimed she was helping her friend, Alexis, who had been very anxious lately. Unbeknownst to Molly, Alexis secured additional meds from two other students. Taken together as a cocktail in the bathroom, she passed out. Luckily, Alexis was found breathing and was currently being treated at a local hospital.

After taking note of the most important part of what he told me so far, Alexis was ok, I took a moment to breathe a sigh of relief before turning my attention back to what the Sergeant was saying. He continued explaining that Molly was very upfront with her role in this and was arrested on site at the request of the school. She was being held at the local police station where they were questioning her further.

I could barely keep up with what he was saying. His voice sounded far away and underwater. I strained to listen, willing him to cut to the chase. What does this all mean? For Molly? For Alexis…I know the Sergeant said she was breathing, but what if something happened at the hospital and she wasn't?

He wouldn't give me any more details. Molly had turned eighteen just two months earlier, and her adult status made her more vulnerable at the hands of the law. It didn't matter that she was arrested from a school where all of the children had a diagnosis and meds were as normalized as a midday meal. It didn't matter to him that they were questioning a child with a mental illness who I was sure was having trouble understanding why she was arrested at all. I wasn't in Molly's head, but I was close to it. I knew she believed she was helping her friend, but that wouldn't, didn't matter here. No, it didn't matter at all. For the first time in my life, I was on the other side of a legal system that I had always believed protected us. In the blink of an eye, we were criminals, and it was clear Molly was guilty until proven innocent.

Finally, my mind snapped into sharp, laser focus on the piece of all this I had control over: taking care of Molly. My dinner time legal training as the daughter of a trial attorney kicked in and I began doing the talking. I made sure she wasn't being questioned without an attorney. I alerted him to her mental status. I got directions to the police station, and I hung up. By the time I clicked goodbye, the mama bear in me had come out of hibernation. I was ready to do all I could to protect Molly.

My first phone call was to Howie. Drawing on a calm efficiency reserved for only the direst of catastrophes, I explained what had happened. He called Jack, our friend and attorney, who was going to meet me at the police station. I followed that call with a more difficult one to my parents who were waiting for a light Friday afternoon lunch. They offered to follow me to the courthouse. Realizing the strength I had mustered could give way at any moment, and understanding my father could speak the language we might need at the police station if we got there before Jack, I welcomed their company.

Snapshots of the past played through my mind as I feared the worst for her future. Molly loved family trips and holidays. Just last fall we went apple picking. She didn't think those sorts of things were too juvenile like many teenagers, and she didn't have a lot of other friends to do things with. Her lack of typical teenage inhibition was contagious and together we jumped onto bales of hay and ate apples straight off the trees until our chins were sticky. She began talking about my grandmother's stuffing months before Thanksgiving, and I usually caught her stealing handfuls before it ever made it into the turkey. Molly loved to help in the kitchen, always ready to crack eggs or help make matzoh balls at Passover. Even though it's hard to allow her chaos into my neatly ordered kitchen, over the years I've learned it's worth it for the momentary closeness. The tighter I held on, the more she slipped away.

Loosening my grip on the steering wheel, I wished it was that easy for me to let go and wondered if things would be different if I did. History had taught me otherwise, but holding on wasn't working anymore either. As I was thinking about other moms who seemed able to let go, my mind wandered back to a friend in Philadelphia.

Like me, Melanie had young children, three under the age of six with one more on the way. We were fast friends, spending as much time together with our kids as without. After tuck in we often met on her porch with other neighborhood moms, talking and drinking wine too late into the night, knowing that waking up would be painful but not caring enough to walk home at a decent hour.

I learned a lot from Melanie. She let her kids play outside in the rain without worrying about muddy footprints, clean up, baths, and all that would follow. I envied her ability to enjoy her kids without worrying that what looked like harmless fun could unravel at any moment. There was one key difference between us. Melanie didn't have a Molly.

But she adored Molly. Always pointing out the good traits, trying to assuage my fears. I was just beginning to put voice to my nagging fears at that time, and she became one of my few confidantes, one of the building blocks of my initial support system.

We talked about parenting challenges and the daily difficulties we faced. We shared a mutual hatred for the witching hours…5–8 p.m. to be exact. For me it was the overall chaos that moved like a tornado through the kitchen, bathroom, and all three bedrooms before I finally collapsed. For Melanie, as she coined it, she never was able to *close the deal*. She'd get her kiddies all fed, bathed, and then felt forever stuck on the next step, bedtime often evading her household way past lights out.

Melanie had a penchant for dropping off small gestures, tokens, just to let me know she was thinking of me. On one morning, I was having trouble keeping my eyes open as I plopped three frozen waffles into the toaster for a quick breakfast before we had to leave for the bus stop. I was paying for a late night on Melanie's porch, our laughs morphing into a serious discussion surrounding my latest concerns about Molly. Most of the time I stayed very focused on what was actionable, what I could do to help her, and just getting through the days. But on Melanie's screened porch in the quiet hours after midnight, I let my guard down to even myself and talked about my deepest fears, about how sick I suspected

Molly really was, and what it really could mean for her and her future. Later, as I walked home way closer to my alarm going off than I should have, I felt cleansed and connected, that underlying dread quieted for the moment.

Later that day a typical Melanie package showed up on our steps. No knock or doorbell announcing her arrival, so quiet that the dogs didn't even bark. I found it there when I left the house with the twins to meet Molly at the afternoon bus. I didn't have time to open it as I had a twin on each hand, so I just kicked it inside our entryway forgetting about it as the witching hours began.

Much later, when the house was quiet again, and I could finally focus on me as a single pronoun, I walked back to the small package. In it was a CD, *Tigerlily* by Natalie Merchant. On it, a single sticky note with the words "Listen to Wonder" written in Melanie's handwriting. I put it into my CD player and on came *Wonder*. The words instantly made me well up with such a torrent of emotions I could almost hear a cork popping. The song is about a mother worried about her daughter and there in the chorus, in a soft, encouraging, folk song style chant, Natalie Merchant assured me, "She'll make her way."

I couldn't get Natalie Merchant and her promise out of my head. I brought *TigerLily* into my car and played Wonder over and over, singing at the top of my lungs with tears streaming down my face. With each chorus I believed the words a little more. It became my anthem.

No song by any other artist since has had as much of an effect as Wonder. Perhaps it was the timing of the gift, given by a friend at just the right moment. To this day, I will find myself humming Wonder or singing "She'll make her way," its effects just as powerful as when Melanie first gifted it to me.

As I continued what seemed like a cross-country trek to

the police station, the reality of this situation set in, and my mind played a tickertape of what ifs.

What if Molly's doctor had never prescribed her meds to take on an as needed basis?

What if I demanded to read Molly's texts and emails as many of my friends did? Would I have intercepted promises for meds that I could have stopped?

What if Molly was a little less naive and could have predicted what her friend was going to do with the meds?

What if I had given in to Molly's daily request to stay home from school today? Would we all be having lunch at the diner?

What if we had never transferred Molly from our local high school?

And the one I just couldn't get out of my head: *what if Alexis isn't okay?*

Windward promised to protect and support the bullied children but had been admitting more troubled children as of late, those that would pay the tuition. Instead of prescriptions, they acquired their drugs with their pocketbooks. During the past year it seemed like Windward had abandoned Molly in more ways than one. Little did I realize this was a foreshadowing of things to come.

Finally, *what if I hadn't answered the phone?*

The power of the phone call itself was immense. It had triggered everything. I thought of Wonder and hoped there was still a chance she'd make her way. As I sped down the road, I instinctively knew we would get through this, but it would be messy. The quiet reprieve of the past months was over.

Molly was released from the police station with a court date, followed by a call from school scheduling a meeting to discuss disciplinary action. There were so many unknowns, and we were powerless to do anything but wait and see.

Wait and see if Molly would be expelled just before graduation.

Wait and see what happened in court.

Wait and see if any of the above affected her college acceptance.

Wait and see if she would graduate high school with her class.

Wait and see how this affected her future overall. At eighteen she aged out of most of her services. We had already lost Marnie, her state-appointed therapist. What else would be taken from us?

After a long weekend filled with anything that would distract us from the elephant in the room, it was a relief when my alarm went off on Monday morning. We were on our way to pick up our attorney, my father, and head to Windward to find out the ramifications of her arrest. It was quiet in the car. Just Molly, Howie, and me. I was lost in my own thoughts. We had talked until we there was nothing more to say and then we talked some more. My eyes had long since dried. Like a wrung-out towel, there was nothing left.

I mechanically kissed my dad's cheek when he got in the car. With his advice, I had presented Molly's case as calmly and thoughtfully as possible on the phone and later in an email to Mr. Bard. We understood the gravity of the situation. What she did was wrong and dangerous. She had been arrested and would pay. As of now we didn't know just how much her mistake would cost.

What was at stake was anything from a slap on the wrist to her college seat. My dad asked how we were all doing and told us it was important we all stay calm and listen to what they have to say. He seemed sure this would result in time served for the suspension she had been in since the incident occurred last week.

At this point I agreed with him. It was unreasonable for

the school to punish Molly more than they had for acting in a way that was in line with her illness. Carrying emergency anxiety meds was as common for her, and many of the kids at Windward, as it was for me to carry around a Tylenol. She was numb to the potential effects on others and sharing it with a friend in need was a natural next step. If it helped her, why wouldn't the meds help her friend? This is how far her immature and naive brain could reason. They accepted Molly at Windward knowing her challenges. Could they really expel her for acting on them?

It started pleasantly enough. Dr. Friedman reviewed what had transpired to be sure we all agreed. "Last week Alexis asked Molly for meds to help with some anxiety she was experiencing. Unfortunately, Molly didn't realize that Alexis also asked some others as well. Alexis ingested all the medications she was given and was found unconscious in the bathroom. I'm happy to report she is home and will make a full recovery."

The conversation continued as to why Molly agreed to give Alexis the meds. He questioned Molly to see if she accepted cash in return. She did not. I watched my dad for signs and could tell by the movement of his jaw he was clenching his teeth trying to let the doctor from Windward do his due diligence. It was painful to stay quiet. His questions seemed very pointed. Finally, I interrupted to explain Molly's naivete and victim role in this whole mess. It was about this time that the tone shifted.

It became clear there was an agenda that hadn't been shared with our side of the table. Mr. Bard shed any more pretenses, explaining this meeting was a formality and Molly's fate already determined.

"My hands are tied. The board *(none of whom were present)* decided in a weekend meeting. Molly cannot to return to Windward. She is expelled."

This was not a meeting. It was not even a trial. It was the delivery of a verdict without any chance to present our case. I didn't even know if our previous discussions and email exchanges had been heard or taken into consideration.

My father started to speak like a lawyer but with the heart of a grandfather. He spoke the words many on both sides of the table were thinking.

"So let me see if I got this straight. A student with a known disability, acts in a manner in line with that disability, as we've established and agreed that Molly did, and you are not suspending her to teach her a lesson, but instead want to expel her, wash your hands of her, for acting out in a way that you promised as an institution to support?"

Silence fell around the room. Even Mr. Bard was momentarily tongue tied before resuming his role as a puppet for the invisible board.

"I'm sorry, but the decision is made."

I wasn't sure I could speak but my mind was reeling. My hands seemed stuck to the papers I had brought, each one of them filled with notes for a discussion that was not going to happen. I fought the urge to stand up and leave and instead tried to focus on what to do next to save Molly's future, wondering desperately if there was a way we could turn this even halfway around. I started to speak to Mr. Bard as if no one else was in the room. Never losing eye contact and trying desperately to control the tension in my jaw. I wondered if anyone could see my neck twitching or hear the tremor in my voice. I spoke, staying focused on keeping my voice from shaking, breaking, or raising in line with what I was feeling inside.

"While I think what you are doing is disappointing, actually absolutely disgusting, and I will always believe you have failed her when she needed you most, my biggest concern is Molly's future. As she is one of the few seniors here admitted to college, I want to be sure this does not jeopardize her admission. How can we make that happen?"

My father smiled at me as if trying to save my daughter's future was groundbreaking. But he jumped right on board to the change in direction.

Then the puppet principal had an idea of his own.

"You can withdraw Molly at any point. And I'm sure we can get a medical exemption for her to be taught at home for the last six weeks. She has always had dual enrollment technically, so she will graduate with her class from her sending school and can even walk with them if she likes."

That sounded almost too good to be true. Something that could protect her future. It also felt like we were shoving their expulsion back at them. I liked that. I stayed calm even though my inner schoolyard girl wanted to stick my tongue out. I needed to be sure.

"If we withdraw Molly, then there will be no expulsion on her record, correct?"

"Yes, that is correct," Mr. Bard confirmed. He smiled as if we were all on the same side. I wanted him to know I still held them accountable. Even if we figured out a way to salvage Molly's future, her present, the end of her senior year, was being taken from her. The punishment didn't seem to fit the crime. My father must have read my mind and started speaking again, this time looking down periodically as if he were reading a closing argument.

"I am glad we were able to figure something out, but I must say I think what you tried to do here is abominable. You have a young lady who before last Wednesday was a student in good standing, had a lead in the play, and was one of your few seniors accepted at what is, I might add, a fine college, and without giving her or her parents any chance to defend her, you just wash your hands of her. No one is saying what happened wasn't horrible, and that she had no role in it. We are saying her intent was to help, and her immaturity and naivete got in the way, which you agree is part of her disability. I think this whole meeting was a sham, and I'm being nice because both my daughter and granddaughter are sitting here." He shot us both smiles and, in that moment, I knew we had gotten over one more crisis.

We figured out the details of gathering her papers and setting up homeschooling in the conference room and finished our conversation about next steps in the parking lot.

Molly, who had been mostly quiet up until this point, asked a few questions about how it would work and seemed generally relieved she wouldn't have to go back to school. Windward rejected her and a person with BPD fears rejection most of all. I tried to focus on the future and a school that accepted her. "The most important thing is that this doesn't affect college and now it won't."

With every crisis comes the after. The aftershock, followed by the aftereffects, followed by just the after—that time when I realize something has changed, shifted permanently. This was no different, and while, even by my life, it was a big one, we still managed to move on into the after.

In this case the aftershock was short lived. I'm not sure I ever really absorbed the fact that my daughter had been arrested and subsequently *(almost)* expelled from her high school just weeks before graduation. It was a complete shattering of my dreams for her. Of course, I recognized we only had the luxury of fighting this fight and being angry for her because of the luck of the outcome. Alexis was okay. Her parents refused contact with us and wouldn't let her speak with Molly, so we were left only knowing what the school told us—that she was getting treatment and was transferring to a different school. But what if the unthinkable had happened and she wasn't okay? It was too much to consider, for her, for her family, and for what it would have meant for Molly.

Luckily, I only had to deal with that scenario in my thoughts. But in those same moments, when trying to visualize Molly's future, the unavoidable roadblocks shine bright. How will she navigate the next judgment call in a world full of them? What if the next big decision, albeit still innocent and without malice, results in someone getting hurt? I didn't have the answers and instead turned to all I really knew—use my coping skills and take it one day at a time.

We focused on the good fortune we were handed when Windward agreed to allow Molly to withdraw and looked forward to the future. I never spoke to anyone at Windward again. Instead, I worked directly with the special needs office at NJ Regional High School. They set up home schooling in a matter of days and before I knew it, we were in a routine. Each morning Molly's assigned tutor came to the house and stayed for three to four hours. Once she left, with almost no nudging from me, Molly easily finished her work in the afternoon. The workload was manageable, almost laughable in the face of what we had dealt with over the years. I wondered ironically why we hadn't done this sooner?

With Leo and Emily at school all day, I suddenly found myself with conflict-free alone time with Molly. During all this she had a scheduled breast reduction surgery to address her growing complaints of back pain, and we spent a lot of time just resting and recovering in the backyard. I tried to direct the conversation forward, to college, and all that she had to look forward to. She was still dealing with all that had happened. Alexis was one of her few friends and they hadn't spoken since that day, and they never would again. Her lead in *Seussical the Musical* was given to someone else, and she was refunded for her ticket to the prom. It seemed so unfair.

Molly had been more of an observer since the arrest, with us taking over, telling her what to say, and mostly telling her to be quiet and let us handle it. When I finally took the time to listen, I hurt for my little girl. These were real losses, and it was a rare moment of clarity for her to voice them. We talked about all of it—what she lost, what could have happened, all we had to be grateful for, and all I hoped she learned from it for her future. It was one of those times that we really connected.

I couldn't fix the past, but I could make what was left special. Her memories of being bullied at NJ Regional High School were still too fresh for her to be comfortable walking at their graduation. So we had our own.

It was a perfect June night, everyone comfortable in the folding chairs set up in the backyard. Our sundresses kept us cool but reminded us we were there for a special occasion. Molly ate up the attention. Her hair and makeup done for the occasion, she greeted the guests as they came. Each one hand chosen for their relationship to our family. Leo and Emily jumped in to help with set up and prepared speeches, determined to celebrate Molly in what they thought was a deserved accomplishment. Leo set up the sound system and was ready to play "Pomp and Circumstance" when signaled. As friends, family, and former therapists who became friends came in through the gate in our backyard, I watched from the top step of the patio. The flowers were all in bloom; their color and sweet fragrance surrounded the folding chairs we had put out, creating an oasis in the middle of our chaos.

The ceremony was short but heartfelt. Several of us spoke, but I remember Marnie's speech the most. After years of counseling, she knew Molly well. While we all told Molly we were proud of her, Marnie also talked about the extra challenges she would face going to college, that she would have to work harder to meet her goals. It wasn't all fluff and maybe that's why it made such an impact.

I tried to soak up every minute. There were so few chances to celebrate things in Molly's life, so many events and crises that overshadowed the good; I wanted to enjoy this moment. Too soon Mark, our friend who also happened to be President of the Board of Education, stood up, and sounding very official, called Molly to the podium where he presented her with a diploma signed by NJR and the Board of Education. Cue Leo. "Pomp and Circumstance" filled the backyard. We all stood up, clapped and cheered as Molly, in *True Molly Fashion*, squealed with delight and threw her cap in the air. Realizing we had given her a moment in the spotlight she earned and watching her make the most of it brought me to tears. I'd cried a lot in the past month, but these were happy tears, and I let them flow as I ran and hugged our graduate.

A week later we found ourselves in court for her hearing. This time the judge heard our case and took time to listen. We explained Molly's punishment to date, her expulsion turned withdrawal and her plans for the future. Once he had all the facts he turned his attention to Molly.

"You understand, young lady, that what you did was wrong and that you and your friend were both very lucky that nothing worse happened?"

Molly nodded, the back of her head looking very small in the courtroom. Two rows back, sitting next to Howie, I wanted to jump in, protect her, yell, *"Of course, we've been through all this, don't you think she paid enough? Let's get on with this and get out of here!"* Instead, I squeezed Howie's hand tighter, my lifeline, so steady. I wondered how this was affecting him. When I looked over and saw him focused on the scene unfolding in front of us like an animal poised to protect, I knew. Together we waited for the sentence.

"Well, Molly, it seems like you understand what you did was wrong, and that you won't do anything like this again. In my opinion, having to leave your school just shy of graduation seems punishment enough for a student in otherwise good standing. And the fact you are headed to college with the support of both your parents makes me feel almost comfortable enough to leave it at that. However, to be sure, you are going to need to complete seventy hours of community service in the next year. You will set that up with the probation officer assigned to you by the court. Good luck, Molly. I hope to never see you here again."

And that was it.

---- CHAPTER THIRTEEN ----

Transitions

> **NOTE:** With Fin's permission, I have used his birth name (Molly) up until this point. Beginning partway through this chapter, he will be referred to as Fin except in flashback.

"I have a secret," Molly said with a mischievous smile. I grabbed Howie's hand in preparation for whatever was coming this time.

"Mom, Dad, I've been thinking about this for a while. You know I've always felt that I'm not in the right body, that I'm not really a girl. Well, I've decided it's time to do something about it."

Shocked into silence once again, my immediate reaction was one I'm glad I kept to myself.

No, this was not something I *knew* she had been feeling her whole life. I'm her mother and would have noticed *something*. This is the same child who slept in ballerina clothes, a girl's girl choosing pink over blue every time.

But I reasoned as I quickly worked through it, it didn't

matter if she was rewriting history, it was what she believed now. I dug into our past for guidance and explanations trying make sense of it all.

I thought back first to Dr. Ellman—knowing he would remind me of how both sexual and gender identity can be on a continuum instead of an either/or choice. Then I thought of Dr. Sanders and our many conversations surrounding Molly's diagnosis of BPD. Among the symptoms associated with BPD, *rapid changes in self-identity and self-image* were one with which we were familiar. Over the years Molly had tried on many personas, embraced lifestyles, experimented with hair color, sexual orientation, even her accent. We learned not to get too attached or to argue when she insisted, *"This is it,"* as the only constant was the next change.

Many times, her shifting identity was tied to her most current obsession. I wondered how much of this decision was influenced by Nathan. She met Nathan in college after struggling some during the first months.

When we dropped her at her freshman dorm, she was excited, ready to take on this new chapter.

"I can't believe I won't be coming home with you. I'm going to live here, back in Philadelphia, now."

It was as if she was saying it out loud to make it real. I always marveled at those times when she sounded so in touch with her emotions—those times of awareness were what I held on to and what had become fewer and farther between in recent years.

"I'm so proud of you for getting yourself to this point. You made this happen and can do whatever you want here. There are so many possibilities. I'm so excited for you. And we're just a short drive away."

"And Daddy's hospital is just up the block!"

We talked about how she and Howie would have dinner,

and I'd come down for a girls' night, while at the same time I hoped that she'd be so wrapped up in college life it would be hard to find time in her schedule. I couldn't see it happening but maybe my intuition was wrong this time.

Sadly, I was right. By the end of that first week, even before classes began, the phone calls started. At all hours of the day and night. Some broke my heart, like during orientation when she had no one to go to meals with. Her roommates knew people and didn't include her. I knew it took time, but I also knew Molly worked in extremes. What was a small setback for others usually became catastrophic for her.

Once again, I was dreading the phone calls. The ring triggered my heart to race out of my chest, my hands shaking as I picked up the phone, never knowing what I'd hear. Hysterical demands to leave, paranoid-like stories of how her roommates were out to get her. Within a week it was clear that the only way to salvage the college experiment at all was to move her dorm. Still trying to fix, I reasoned if roommates were the problem, let's remove the problem.

I got busy on the phone with housing, pulling out all the stops, flaunting her diagnosis, concerns for her mental stability and her safety. I appealed to them as a mother. I cried real tears as I pleaded her case.

"I don't want her to fail so fast. She needs a success she can build on, not a failure that could set the tone for her future."

Underneath it all was what I couldn't say out loud. I didn't want her home. Even though I hated the phone calls, the distance made it easier. Just a wall between our rooms was nowhere near enough, and I was desperate not to move backward. I didn't have an alternate post-grad plan. I was determined to make this one work.

Molly doubled down on the calls and desperate pleas. I

tuned her out, sure I could fix this. Finally…success! I found the only single left on campus and moved her into it the next week. Gone were the helpful students and large bins. Like pack mules, we lugged the contents of her room across campus. I set her up in her new studio on a top floor with a beautiful view overlooking downtown Philly. Before I left, we talked about fresh starts, all she liked about school, her classes, and living on her own. I was smiling as I drove over the Ben Franklin bridge back to New Jersey. She had a new start and seemed quietly resigned to try.

Over the next few months, late night emergency calls stopped. I went down to visit a few times and slept in her room. Each time cleaning it from top to bottom while she sat on her bed *exhausted*. Like when she was younger and I had to continuously put her homework back in front of her before she'd do it, I hoped by showing her how to clean, keep a home, organize her work, over and over again, it would eventually sink in. It never did with her homework, but I naively thought age and time would make a difference.

You only see what you choose to see. Looking back, I wanted this to work so badly. A pivotal point that set her on the right path. What path? To a career? To happiness? Both? I didn't really know, but I kept doing what I did best, pointing her there anyway. With every negative I pointed out a positive. Every time she begged to come home, I told her to stick it out. But Molly is tenacious—once she decides something is not going to work, she sticks to it.

It was easy to ignore the signs, and it was difficult to know what a normal period of adjustment was versus red flags we shouldn't ignore. Molly lived in extremes and not all of them became crises. Over the years it became hard to tell the difference until it was right there in front of me. Maybe I became dulled to signs, the distance making it easier to pretend.

By winter we couldn't ignore it anymore. She was missing classes, the work was piling up as high as the excuses, claiming everything from illness to her professors' unavailability or refusal to honor her accommodations. I couldn't fix this—Molly was an adult and, except for paying the bills, no one at the University would talk to me about academics.

Molly was sinking. Reasoning was off the table. She insisted everyone was against her. The professors, the students, and even the people in the special needs office. Slowly her willingness to try my suggestions went from begging to come home to threats of self-harm.

We had to step in, and I reached deep into our history of Philadelphia to someone who would talk to us and who we knew could help. Dr. O'Connor was a short train ride away and was willing to meet with his former patient. We made a deal. She agreed to stay for the remainder of the year, trying her best, seeing Dr. O'Connor regularly. We agreed if she was still unhappy at the end of the school year, she didn't have to return.

Molly started taking the train to Bryn Mawr and sounded better each week. She enjoyed exploring Philadelphia, finding freedom in being able to get on the train and leave when she wanted.

Then she met Nathan.

At first, I thought he was the answer. A friend, maybe even a boyfriend. She only needed one to counter her isolation. Someone to go out with. A segue to the rest of the social scene on campus. I really believed that was all it would take.

And for a while Nathan sounded great. Like many others before him he went from a new friend to an obsession overnight. Our calls were filled with his name.

"Nathan saved me a seat in class."

"Nathan smiled at me and looked at me with his blue eyes. I melted."

"Nathan walked me home after class."

If he was the reason she was going to class and engaging in college, who was I to argue? I asked more questions, trying to learn more about her latest idol. Knowing from experience, she would embrace all of him. I needed to know what we were in for.

Nathan was somewhere between a sophomore and a junior. I never quite got a straight answer. He lived in a fraternity house and seemed to have some other friends. He was in one of her classes and saved her a seat every day. They talked about everything. They went together to a few parties on campus and then ventured to South Street in Philly. Nathan introduced her to his world of cross dressing, drag queens, and the LGBTQ community. Everyone she met had felt as outcast as her at some point and welcomed her with open arms. She was hooked. And I was happy she found a friend and a community.

Within weeks she knew everything about Nathan. His favorite colors, foods, clothing—you name it, she knew it. And it didn't stop there; it was like she absorbed him, would have become him if given the chance. His interests became hers, his fights and causes hers too. Almost overnight, Molly knew the names of all the pop culture drag queens, became a daily devotee of *RuPaul's Drag Race*, and became a regular at the drag bars in South Philly.

She didn't dress in drag, but instead became a friend to many of the performers, finding a niche in learning to dress them, picking out costumes and applying makeup. She was happy, calling often to regale us with stories of her nights out and new friends. She was reinvented. And she rewrote her own history to fit. She had *always* loved drag, been interested in cross dressing, and anything else Nathan.

I didn't know what to think. She was happy, but I was unsure. I was uncertain if Nathan loved her the same way she obviously loved him. I wasn't even sure she knew she loved him. But she was away. She was at college and if she was to grow, I needed to let her try these things out. I watched from the wings as much as I could but ready with the net should she fall.

The emergency calls were replaced by happy, mostly one-way chats. I asked with some apprehension how classes were going, and she always brushed me off with a *fine* before continuing with how beautiful Nathan looked in the red dress she picked out for him the night before. If I had listened closely, perhaps I would have heard the warning not to push further about school, but I chose not to. I was enjoying our distance and the happiness she was finding in this new world. It was easier, and I hoped she was sliding by academically.

As the weather warmed, I knew I had to re-visit our agreement. I pinned too much hope on Nathan. That he alone would be enough to keep her in college. But she stood firm. Although she sounded happy when we talked about her nightlife, she finally told us her life outside of Nathan was the same. It was like a switch flipped as she piled on the excuses and reasons for her failing grades in most classes

"Professor X hates me."

"Professor Y never answers my emails."

"Professor Z grades me unfairly because he doesn't like me."

When I pressed, she got more defensive, pointing over and over to how college is just not for her, and we promised she could leave after this year. I pointed out the deal was that she tried, but I was grasping at straws. I pushed harder and she pushed back. She had an answer for everything. She'd be friends with Nathan forever, she promised, and he agreed college wasn't for her. Then she told me he was probably dropping out too. I tried making her look forward, reminding her she was an adult and needed to do something.

"What are you planning to do?" I asked, not expecting an answer.

"I want to go to beauty school so I can do the makeup for *RuPaul's Drag Race*." After rolling my eyes, glad she couldn't see me on my end of the phone, I tried to see it from her point of view. College wasn't for everyone. I knew that now. Makeup had a future, and she had always been good at it. I began fast forwarding. She could work on movie sets; my brother could help get her a job...maybe this wasn't such a bad idea.

Howie went alone to move her out. He described the scene to me that night in a hushed voice once Molly was settled in the next room.

"I couldn't believe what I was seeing. There was so much garbage I could barely see the floor. Every surface was covered with trash, dirty clothes, dirty dishes, open food containers, you name it. It smelled as bad as it looked. I don't want to think about it. Stacy, I can't believe she was living there. I know having her home won't be easy, but we really don't have a choice."

Nathan continued to be Molly's focus throughout the next couple of years. Her guiding light around which she made all critical life decisions. It was clear she was in love with a fantasy she could never have. He was gay.

Next up, beauty school. She made some friends, dressed the part, and seemed happy. Until she wasn't. Like everything else, the novelty wore off, and the demands, however small in my eyes, became too much. Again, I pushed, demanding she cross the finish line, betting again that if she'd just finish and get a job this would be it. I should never go to Vegas.

Beauty school turned out to be a $16,000 blip, although she made it to graduation. We were all there, Howie, the twins, and my parents. And we watched her walk down the makeshift graduation aisle at Paul Mitchell School to her classmates clapping. Like in our backyard, *(was it only two years earlier?)* she was glowing. I let myself feel the pride—kvelling we call it. I didn't get a chance much with her. I didn't let myself except for the big things. It was like a learned aversion. If I got too comfortable, the seat would only be pulled out from under me.

It didn't take long for the next shoe to fall. At our graduation dinner she announced she would not be taking the certification test required to get any jobs in the field. There was no arguing with her. She was an adult. We couldn't force her and didn't have the energy to try.

We were at a crossroads that could easily become a standoff. College out. Vocational school, a trade, a failure. Now what? It was hard enough having her home while going to beauty school, but I had held on to graduation day like a life raft. Now I felt the air flowing out of it.

We demanded she work if she was living home, and she began a series of short-lived jobs. Her moods changed as quickly as her employment. I never knew what I'd find when I came home. It wasn't long before I felt like a prisoner in my own home and found myself making any excuse I could to stay away.

"I'm staying at work late."

"I'm going to the supermarket."

"I have a doctor's appointment."

"I'm meeting a friend for dinner."

Her temper continued to flair unexpectedly. We didn't

know what would trigger her. Something as small as asking to change the channel could send us all to our bedrooms for the night.

And then there was that fateful New Year's Eve. I don't remember how it started, but I remember how it ended.

"911. What's your emergency?"

"My child. She broke a window and now she's threatening to jump out of it. I'm worried she's going to hurt herself and maybe us."

The police came and, after some coaxing, took her to the hospital. Within two hours *(just shy of midnight)* she was released. The hospital staff brushed off our concern about bringing home someone who was so violent just hours earlier. They seemed more interested in clearing house before the ball dropped. I wondered where in the parenting manual was how to handle all of this, and as December 31st came to a close, I thought back to New Year's Eves past, of my younger self, always full of hope for the future. I thought about my Molly, with her wispy, blonde hair and electric eyes and wondered where I failed.

Today's announcement snapped me back to the present, wishing for a parenting manual that covered *this*.

"I'm a boy and starting now I'm going to live like one. I'm changing my name to Fin. I know this may be hard for you, but it is who I am, and I hope you will accept it."

She could sound so mature and diplomatic when she wanted to, but I knew that last line was both a question and a challenge. She stopped and looked at us expectantly. We didn't say anything. We were letting her finish and gathering our thoughts.

"You have another son!" she filled the silence with an excited laugh as if it were a gender reveal party.

Fin began living his life as a man with our support. While

the BPD symptom *a shifting sense of identity* initially gave me pause and I wondered if he'd change his mind in line with BPD, I quickly learned it didn't matter. If transitioning made him happier, and helped him become independent, I was all in.

Fin spent the next few years moving further away from us both physically and figuratively. I learned my pronouns and to respect his wishes.

After the college experiment and beauty school rebound, Fin's life became a series of crises, tried and failed attempts at new starts, more experiments. It was as if he were working his way through textbook BPD symptoms:

Unstable, intense relationships,

Idealizing someone one minute and then believing the person doesn't care or is against them,

Suicidal thoughts or threats of self-harm in response to fear of someone leaving them or of separation,

Distorted self-image,

Mood swings.

At the center of each crisis was a relationship that gathered strength at breakneck speed and broke up, leaving damage that felt like a category five storm. Then a new one, fresh and ready to tackle it. Unfortunately, Fin carried very few lessons forward and continued to make the same mistakes over and over. I began to feel more like a bank teller than a mom, with him refusing advice until an emergency, and then calling to demand money to get him out of whatever mess he found himself in.

The first one surrounded Nathan. Against our advice, he moved in with Nathan and two others in an apartment just outside Philadelphia. Again, *this was it.* This was Fin's dream come true. He was going to live with Nathan and move forward with transitioning. While I didn't agree with this move, it was so much easier when he wasn't home. We filled his car with used tables, chairs, plates, cups, and anything else I could find.

Barely any time passed before the late-night phone calls started.

History had taught me that as soon as Fin sensed rejection, no matter how small, the relationship was ending. He just didn't have the tools to work through disagreements, and the reality of a rejection was too much for him to handle. He'd rather sabotage a relationship then wait for a rejection. I began the painful torture of waiting, and when this one rolled in, it was a big one.

I'm not sure what time of day it began, but it was a series of phone calls of him hyperventilating in high pitched sobs that Nathan wanted him out and he didn't want to leave.

"Mom, he doesn't want me here anymore. I don't know what I did, but he said I have to leave. Can I please come home?"

Nathan yelling in the background. More sobbing.

My knees suddenly weak, I sat down to think. Desperate to save the situation, to keep him in Philly both to avoid another failure and to stop at all costs another homecoming, I tried to help him work it out. I even asked to talk to Nathan. But when Nathan got on the phone, gone was the soft spoken, awkward, feminine manchild I had spent so much time with over the past two years. An aggressive and threatening Nathan told me in no uncertain terms that Fin was crazy, and while he will always love him, they can't live together. When I pointed out that Fin had paid rent, appealing to fairness, and yes, the legal reality of what he was doing, his true colors came out.

"I don't care about your cheap Jew threats. I want him out."

That was the last I ever spoke to Nathan. Fin moved home, and within days he was defending Nathan, blaming himself and ready to go back if Nathan called. Fin will do anything to salvage a relationship with one of his obsessions rather than accept rejection and admit failure.

With Fin home again we were right back in it. So many symptoms on display—quick to anger, violent and frequent mood swings—we were all tiptoeing around trying to avoid a fight.

The growing distance between us became a rift. Fin was always ready to pounce. His thinking was disorganized, bouncing between mourning the loss of an imagined romance to blaming us for the choices he now faced. He moved between the couch and his room, food containers and dirty clothes, and a tell-tale stench marking his whereabouts. I chose my battles carefully, allowing him to almost live in his room. The tension was thick, and when I attempted to cut it, I became the unwitting target of the next attack. Once again, Fin was ruling the house.

I couldn't figure this one out. This couldn't be it. The rest of his and my life. Under his reign I felt like there was a vice on my head at all times, afraid of what I'd find every time I left my room. I wasn't looking for the fairytale anymore—just something a little lighter than the horror show we were living in. We all deserved better. Tired of walking on eggshells in my own home, I sat down facing him on the L of the couch where we used to sit for family therapy, and asked point blank what his plans were.

He continued staring at the TV, RuPaul or one of her descendants was singing and dancing. I stood up and grabbed the remote.

"What?" He looked at me innocently, genuinely shocked at my frustration.

I tried to tread softly. Eyes on the goal. Ask, don't tell, I repeated in my head. "What are your plans, Fin? You can't just sit here every day."

Frustrated eye roll, but thankfully, no explosion. I went a little further.

"You have to get a job. Dad and I are happy to help..."

"I. Don't. Want. Your. Help!" he screamed.

He was up off the couch, knees bent and staring through me. In a sudden standoff, I stood up too, every muscle tensed, waiting for the next move.

"I am trying to get a job. I left Wawa because the manager wouldn't use my pronouns. She hated me and just took me off the schedule because I'm trans. She said it was because I was late and didn't show up for a shift, but I know better. And at Acme, the deli guy kept calling me Molly even though I told him over and over again my name is Fin. And now with my back, I have pain down my legs and can barely walk sometimes. I think I have a slipped disc. I asked Dad to get me an MRI, but he just ignored me like usual. That's just like him. I'm not his precious Leo and Emily, your perfect children. I'm the fuck up. You never really wanted me..."

My head was spinning. And whether he was trying or not, it worked. I was thrown off topic, the familiar tug of guilt. It was true Leo and Emily were easier, but did I love them more? I was certainly coming to the realization that life was easier when he wasn't here. What did that say about me? He got me where it still hurt.

I took a deep breath and answered as carefully and truthfully as I could.

"Fin, you know that's not true. We love all of you equally but differently. We just want you to be happy, and sitting around all day is unhealthy for all of us."

He knew he had me. Appealing to my affection deflected the real topic. He was an artist at creating a chaotic web of disorganized thinking and then catching you in it. If I didn't get back on track, we would never get to the job, never move forward.

"Oh yeah...you've always loved them more. I'm nothing but a fuck up. I failed out of college and that's all you and Daddy care about. That's all you ever cared about!" Frustration and tears took over.

Hearing these words from any other child, or even adult, would make me stop and think. But coming from Fin, it was pure manipulation and like a yo-yo the weak moment was quickly shed. Manipulation was classic for BPD. I sometimes didn't see it, but on this day I did. I knew the best way to shock him back to reality was to be clear and direct, leaving no room for interpretation.

"Oh, stop it Fin. You know better than that. You know we don't care what you do. But you are an adult, and if you are living here you need to get a job or make plans to move out. Sitting around is unacceptable."

"I know, Mom, and I'm working on it."

I jumped at this bit of news like a fish going for the bait.

"Oh...tell me more."

Without realizing it, we both sat down again as he told me he had made a friend online though a friend from high school. He was going that weekend to meet this new friend at a concert.

"Where is this person from?"

"Arkansas."

Fin moved to Arkansas shortly after this new friend told him about a job there. Fin met Zaq a few months later. While Zaq wasn't why Fin moved to Arkansas, he was, and still is, the reason Fin stays. At the time they met, Fin was living alone, in between jobs once again. We were helping him again. Our contact reduced to demands for cash so much so that I felt like nothing more than an ATM to him. Yet, he was far away, and our life was lighter with the distance. The tradeoff was worth it for the peace I found on most days.

We first met Zaq when they visited together. That was a good visit. They were like fish out of water in New Jersey but seemed happy together. He used the right pronouns but referred to Fin as his *little lady* and I fleetingly tried to figure it all out. I understood the mechanics but was a generation away from understanding the fluid nature of gender and admired their easy acceptance and understanding of all the nuances. However, looking at Zaq, he seemed more play a game of pool with me, man's man, than someone touting gender fluidity at a rally. I wondered how he would deal when Fin began the hormones he was researching. But I shelved that thought

We visited Fin in Arkansas once. We arrived full of plans to take him and Zaq out to dinner, take him shopping, and let him show us anything he wanted.

We got into town on a Friday night and Fin told us Zaq wasn't feeling well so they would see us the next day. I tried to protest, suggest Fin meet us anyway, but Howie's touch on my shoulder while I was talking reminded me not to push. Instead, I sent our best and told him we were looking forward to seeing them the next day.

After dinner and drinks at a quiet restaurant in downtown, I felt better. I even checked in with Fin and made plans to drive the half hour to his place with lunch the next day. Fin explained that Zaq didn't like restaurants, and we wanted to spend time with the latest person that had become the center of Fin's life.

The next morning, we got up as planned and drove to the college town surrounding Arkansas University. The heat reminded me school was on break and explained the sleepiness of the town. We found a pizza place open and placed a too large order so Fin would have leftovers to fill his fridge.

Once back in our car, as Howie put the directions into Waze, I tried Fin to let him know we were on our way. No answer. I tried again. Still no answer. I texted. No answer. We looked at the GPS and saw it would take 40 minutes to get there so we headed out, reasoning he would wake up as we drove.

As we drove out of the city, the towns became progressively more spread out. The homes grew smaller and more rundown and seemed to stand out like blemishes scattered across the Arkansas landscape. Uncared for, they seemed almost angry in their neglect. Difficult to get any reception, the only sound in the car was my phone repeatedly going straight to voicemail.

We found Fin's apartment, the top floor of a rundown house on a road just behind the main road of a town that was barely a town. I jumped out of the car as soon as Howie parked and ran up the back steps, releasing the tension of hours of unanswered calls before once again buttoning it up in the hopes of a good visit.

When our knocks became bangs, we finally heard footsteps and an angry yet familiar, "what do you want?" Relief he was okay flooded my veins and was just as quickly replaced by annoyance at his lack of consideration for our plans, our visit, and us in general.

But then I saw him, and I remembered my expectations are often born out of my personal history; my reality was in front of me, and the two did not match. Fin was wearing men's boxer shorts and a man's robe that he was barely holding closed over his breasts still scarred from his breast reduction. Tattoos, some professional and some poor attempts at home work, were scattered on his arms, torso and legs. Remnants of his cutting phase from high school still scarred much of his body.

I forced myself to look past his scars and mine and search for my child who obviously still needed us very much. It was both easier and harder now that for most of the time he was hundreds of miles away. His distance gave me the strength to build boundaries designed to keep him out when I needed space and to let him in when he needed me. This visit was planned, and I thought I came prepared. But I never really am. I arrived much like a parent at sleep away camp visiting day. Ready for a child longing for maternal love and attention only to be met with the rejection of a troubled mind looking to be saved in all the wrong ways.

He let us in with a grunt, as if it were a big favor, forgetting his promise to meet for lunch, and barely remembering we had driven eight hours to get here. He plopped onto the worn couch sounding as out of breath as a person double his age. The smell in the apartment spoke volumes, telling me he was still smoking, the cat litter needed to be taken out, and he himself needed a good shower. But still I trudged on, hoping somehow to turn this around.

He was silent. Challenging our dedication to the visit and maybe to him all together by lighting a cigarette right in front of us. His lips forming a smirk around the homemade cigarette, a *rollie*, told me we should leave. But I knew if we left, we were abandoning the visit and driving straight home, and I just couldn't do that. Howie busied himself with bringing in the food we almost forgot in the car.

Like a television mom I brightly ignored the scene around me describing all the goodies we brought and putting them away in the otherwise empty refrigerator. I glanced at the sink, noting dishes and containers piled high, overflowing onto the counter, the height of the discarded meals directly proportioned with the depths he seemed to be sinking in right now.

As I worked, I tried to engage him, finding things, however mundane to chatter on about. The mountains, our hotel, where we ate, the cute college town. I knew how desperate I sounded but I didn't care. The silence was too hard to take. As I kept talking, I got more and more frustrated. I changed tactics, instead questioning him. "What's the matter? You seem so upset."

"Nothing's the matter, okay? I just don't feel well."

"Where's Zaq?"

I hit a nerve. He leaned forward, balling up all the tension that had been building and threw it at me full force.

"He's not here, Mother! Don't you get it? We're done. And it's your fault. He didn't want to see you and I tried to force him and now he won't talk to me. And I don't know what to do. I don't know what to do without him. I don't want to do anything. I just want to get him back. He's my everything. Nothing else matters without Zaq. He is the best thing that ever happened to me..."

And there it was. Zaq had replaced Nathan, who had replaced many before him. Some real relationships, some celebrity idols as far back as Justin Bieber when he was a she and barely a teeny bopper. Each one not just a crush, but an obsession he was willing to give up everything for, and the apartment I was sitting in that day in Arkansas told me the stakes were not just threats anymore.

Zaq and Fin made up later that day and many times after that. At first, they seemed happy. Fin's phone calls were full of idyllic stories of trips to a nearby lake, meeting and spending time with Zaq's family, and building a home together in a house Zaq built with his own hands. Zaq, he claimed, was a contractor, but because of multiple health issues was, at twenty-nine, dependent on his disability check to survive.

Fin absorbed Zaq and his lifestyle. It wasn't long before Fin claimed more and more reasons he couldn't work. Without medical proof to back up his physical complaints, Fin never qualified for disability. Real or imagined illnesses and transphobia, a reality where he lives, were his reasons for remaining unemployed. Zaq and the area they lived in both welcomed and rejected him. It allowed him to live on the edge of society, just rejecting him enough that he had an excuse for remaining stagnant. He seemed to be sinking deeper, almost comfortably into a lifestyle that left him constantly on the brink of homelessness.

We were his only source of income and so our ATM status intensified. While the distance made it easier, the extremes felt like I was going through my own climate crisis. One phone call left me hopeful, thoughts of Fin in a relationship, talks of engagement, and he was happy. Another, with him begging for money, made me ruthless in my parenting, creating budgets, even a contract, and promises of deadlines that we never kept. The hope, and my deepest fear overriding my ability to cut him off completely.

When it comes to Fin my deepest darkest fear is one I allude to often but never voice. I am afraid he will die. I do not see his life as sustainable, and it terrifies me.

Almost everything I do with regard to Fin is, in some part, so that I know I did everything in my power to give him the opportunity to make a life for himself. It's getting harder with each passing year. Tough love has become the cliche we return to again and again. With tough love we are removing his supports, making it harder for him to live comfortably without a job. But, I am conflicted; by keeping him comfortable he has shown he will not move forward. What if removing those supports doesn't push him forward but closer to where I cannot go?

I don't know the answer. I only know that I can't just keep him alive in the steady state he is in. It is beating me down. I've spoken to all the professionals, gathered more input than I know what to do with, and the consensus is that we are doing the right thing. I hope pushing him will make him more independent—and ultimately make us able to have a healthy relationship.

But if they're all wrong, I am the one who caused it. We could just continue to support him and let him exist. I don't know which is better. And I won't until it's too late.

Then there were phone calls that left me winded and shaking, or worse, put me into what felt like a waking nightmare as our worlds, limping along miles away, collided when I least expected it. This one began in the middle of the night. I was sleeping soundly when I rolled over, heart already pounding, as I instinctively picked up the ringing phone. My sleepy hello was met with hiccup-filled hysterics. "Mama, he threw me out, it's over. I need to come home."

Shedding my sleep, I sat up, still whispering, the room only lit by the glow from my cell phone. Trying to keep my voice from matching his hysterics, I began peppering him with questions.

"Where are you?"

"Are you safe?"

"What happened?"

I learned he was in his car just outside his house. This fight, though I never learned the exact cause or topic, was the finale in what had been building through a series of episodes.

Fin stopped short of telling me what had happened up until now and turned his attention to Zaq. His voice became muffled as he dropped the phone into a pocket or bag but left the line open. I could hear the fight unfolding like a show. No longer part of the conversation, I was its sole audience.

"Zaq, I love you, why don't you love me anymore?" Fin whimpered, the pleading in his voice loud and clear. Then the sound of the car door slamming followed by his steps climbing toward Zaq.

Zaq's voice came across loud and clear, deep and husky, rising in volume to match his three hundred plus pound size.

"I don't love you. You hear? I never loved you. Now get off of my property or I will call the cops and have you hauled away."

Worried where this was going, I woke up Howie and turned the lights on in the bedroom. Panicking, I started yelling into the phone.

"Fin, turn around and walk away." Louder and louder until he finally took me out of his pocket. His receding steps. A car door slamming. A shuddering sigh. He was back in the car.

"Mama, what should I do? I have nowhere to go. Can I please come home? I promise it will be different. I'll go into a program and get help. I promise. Please. I'll move back home. Get a job. Go on medication. I need my family. I just need my mommy."

Tears welled up, a slick sheen of sweat formed between my palm and my phone. I began to break. The boundary I had begun to put into place, trying to force his independence, crumbled under the weight of my fears for his safety. Hands shaking, I passed the phone to Howie, and repeated over and over, "I don't know what to do. He can't come back here. I don't know what to do."

He took the phone from me at the same moment Emily,

home for summer break, opened the door a crack, peeking into our bedroom, her need to know what was going on equally matched by her desire not to.

"Is Fin okay?"

I lifted my arm waving her toward the bed where she fit between us like a missing puzzle piece, her head resting on my chest immediately calming the pounding that had set in.

We listened to Howie's side of the call.

"Are you safe now?"

"If you don't feel safe, drive to a police station."

"We need to get you somewhere safe tonight so you can sleep and we can figure things out in the morning."

As I lay there straining to hear Fin, I was having a parallel conversation with myself.

We don't have a choice. He has to come back here. We will find him a place to stay.

Maybe this is time will be different.

I just have to set it up with the right rules and stick to them.

I will find him an apartment, get him into therapy; he'll even find a job.

We can do this.

I bent down to kiss the top of Emily's head and rubbed her shoulder. We shivered even though the air conditioner was barely cooling our room from the summer heat wave.

I glanced at the clock. The late hour helped me make my decision. I turned my head to Howie and reached for the phone.

"He needs to come home. I'll get him money to go to a hotel tonight. You go to sleep. You have to operate tomorrow."

This was our well-rehearsed dance. Our taking turns leading while the other regroups. Our saving grace. After years of practice, we balanced each other out in a way that only we understood.

He nodded at me as he handed me the phone and rolled over, reclaiming his sleep. I told Fin the plan as Emily and I relocated to her bedroom.

He came home for the day, they made up, and he left and went back to life in Arkansas with Zaq as if nothing happened. Until the next call.

"Mama, can you send me extra money this month."

"Why, are you in trouble?"

"Can you? I need extra money this month. I need it now. I'm moving to Vermont."

"Fin, what's going on, is everything okay?"

"This is it. Zaq doesn't love me anymore. He said I've made him a laughingstock in town and left. He's not coming back until I move out. So I'm going to Vermont. Amy is there and she has a place set up for me to move into."

Then he burst into tears.

I let him cry and tried to just be a mom for a bit. We talked about how it is painful to be rejected and relationships ending are always hard and all the fixings that go along with that conversation. He let me mother him. The irony of how a painful moment in Fin's life felt so good for me was not lost. For a moment, my hunger to connect was fed. He listened as I told him no one should treat him poorly, and even if it hurt, I'd rather him leave than hold on just because he was afraid of being alone. My heart ached for Fin, yet I didn't want it to end. I even wanted more. My guard was down and my heart took over.

"Before you drive all the way to Vermont, you should come here. You can regroup, get your car inspected, and we can get you the right clothes for Vermont winters." I should know better.

"Okay," Fin said in his newly testosterone-assisted voice that suddenly sounded too small for the two hundred pound body it was coming from. Any trace of a southern twang he usually flaunted gone.

"I'll let you know exactly when I'll get there, and you'll send me money for gas?"

"Of course." Our promise for no extra money each month gone with my boundaries. I was fully in it.

We hung up full of I love yous and call if you need mes.

He called the next day just to tell me he decided to go straight to Vermont. He was there barely a week when they made up. His daily calls and texts dwindled again until…nothing. Our increasingly urgent texts went unanswered until finally, a call.

"Hi Mom, so Zaq and I worked it out, but I still want to come visit. I need to get my car inspected."

I tried to hold onto the pre-Vermont connection, but it was gone. His voice was larger, the Arkansan twang was back.

It's funny how the rollercoaster just kept coming for us. Up and down. Crisis to crisis. We were only along for the ride. But what I only realized in hindsight is that I was learning. Learning that each crisis, visit, argument, will pass, and learning how to cope with them while they're happening. While the shoes kept falling, they stopped knocking me down quite as hard or for as long as they once had. I was learning not to expect them to stop falling. That was a child's fairytale. I just wanted them to lighten up so I could find happiness and peace in the in between.

Knowing Fin was safe, I breathed easily and began preparing for him to visit. It was like preparing for a race—considering all the potential pitfalls and planning strategies for success, for finishing. The better prepared I was, the higher the chances were for emerging unscathed. Preparing in this way took very little emotional investment either. Instead of excitement building as it did when Leo or Emily came to visit, the dread accompanying a visit from Fin could become paralyzing. Going through the motions with an almost comfortable detachment was a form of self-preservation that made me feel safe and calm.

First, I went into what was his room and removed the beautiful white quilt that I'd bought when I converted it into a guest room. I did so about a year ago, finally taking the time to clean out the filth. Piles of junk had filled every corner. Different than hoarding, Fin didn't save, he just used things and moved on. His life could be studied in layers around the room much like the rings of tree. The deepest layers held papers from his school years. Yearbooks, teen books, journals all mixed in with clothes and underwear he hadn't worn for years. As I sorted through, I read some of the journals, searching for and finding the little girl who had lived here. She was at times full of hope, her intelligence shining through both in the language she used and the insight she seemed to have. I also felt her pain during her teen years as she was bullied. I noted how her handwriting changed, becoming larger, more frenzied, almost desperate. In her later journals, her thoughts were angrier and more chaotic, the pen often making holes in the paper. When I couldn't take it anymore, I boxed up the yearbooks and books for him to have one day, knowing he would probably never take them. The next layers reflected the past four years of visits. The clothes grew larger and more masculine, even some of Howie's mixed in. Framed pictures of Fin as a girl from his childhood had been ripped from the walls, leaving angry holes, and thrown into the pile joined by any other decorations he thought feminine. Finally, a layer of cat litter seemed to cover the room from when he "hid" his cats in the closet during his most recent visit.

The result was a welcoming room that I decorated in spa-like neutrals. A white quilt, repurposed window treatment, a comfy chair from our room, and a dresser from Wayfair now welcomed guests. I even had a drawer of sample toiletries I collected over the years in case anyone forgot anything. I think I tried to make it extra welcoming and serene to counter the chaos that was there before.

As I got ready for Fin's visit, I tried to remove anything that could be ruined. The white comforter went first, replaced by a brown quilt from the basement. I put the decorative pillows in my closet, made sure there were no offensive family pictures, and laid out a fresh toothbrush and the other toiletries remembering, how he loved to take baths, playing with lotions and various skin products. As I admired my handiwork, I let myself hope that maybe the calmness would help him. Maybe it is what he needed. Maybe it would be a good visit. Maybe...

CHAPTER FOURTEEN

A Soft Landing

"How about snuggling on the couch and watching a movie?" I asked in my best mommy voice.

All three kids stopped in their tracks. Even Molly, who was always moving the fastest, always the hardest to stop once she started something.

"Yay!" they cried in unison.

I set up the movie and turned to sit on the couch. They were sitting three in a row, Leo hanging off one arm of the sofa, Molly lying on the other, and Emily between them, still holding her Barbie. I wanted to lie down.

Hmmm…

"Everyone up. We're going to pile on Mommy and really snuggle."

At ages three, three and six, they were young enough not to realize that I was angling to be horizontal, unencumbered by their small bodies. Once I was set up and comfortable, I gave the signal.

"Okay, everyone. Find a spot."

In seconds Leo was crouched between the crook of my knees and the couch, Molly was perched on my right hip, and Emily backed into me, fitting like a spoon. I clicked the remote and as the opening credits started to scroll, I felt a sense of peace come over me. Everyone was occupied, safe, and happy. The connection of their little bodies to my own seemed to fill me in a way I really needed on that cold winter's day, ready to start again when the closing credits inevitably made their way across the screen.

Perfection.

These memories from a simpler time still feed me when I need it most. But trauma is funny. It numbs you from the inside out. Some moments frozen like specimens waiting for closer examination. Others rewritten in a way that's easier to digest. And still others become blurry as if you are watching a horror movie from between the gaps in your fingers.

When we're young, we see the world in black and white. Rules comfortably define boundaries, creating order. We grow within that order, placing our thoughts, our actions, and those of the people around us neatly into categories: good and bad, right and wrong. Whatever nomenclature we attach remains crystal clear until it doesn't anymore. Seemingly suddenly, black and white blurs into gray, revealing all the shades in between. The full rainbow is both beautiful and frightening. Clarity adds dimension and finding your truth becomes more challenging. You must search for it. As your mind opens so does your heart, ready to fill with acceptance and gratitude.

I always thought it would be different. I hoped. But it never was. All I could do was prepare, and then dig my heels in to get through it. Protecting myself by removing any kind of emotion from Fin's visits has become almost automatic but not something I ever get used to. It is not who I am and feels stiff, unnatural, yet safe and comfortable in an alarmingly too familiar way.

I got ready for this visit by reviewing the boundaries I'd set up and making empty promises to myself about maintaining them. Like a sleepwalker I go through the motions remaining as numb as possible. Thinking how sad it is to feel the need to lock up valuables, change the garage codes, and replace the new white quilt with an old worn-out comforter is just too painful.

Before I knew it, he arrived. Like a tornado he blows into the house, his cone of destruction immediately creating chaos. The air feels heavier and I'm almost dizzy trying to maintain a semblance of order. He arrives mid-sentence, his own nerves palpable. The sadness at our mutual discomfort blows through me. His words don't make sense. He rambles about nonsensical topics without taking a breath until I am trapped in his turmoil. I take a breath and try to remain calm. Deep in his illness he personifies his chaos by wearing dirty clothes that don't fit and carrying all his belongings as if in a shelter. He moves continuously, leaving a trail of clothing in his path. As his tales spin faster, I am reminded of how much his mental illness has robbed him of. I feel the familiar pit in my stomach, and the pain I work so hard to keep at bay is once again front and center. My eyes fill as I think of the little girl who used to stroke my cheek when she thought I fell asleep in her bed reading one more chapter of *Junie B. Jones*. And I hope. Maybe he will remember too and come back to me.

We sit down to the takeout boxes of Thai food now cold on the table. He opens his and without a thank you begins shoveling food into his mouth without taking a breath. I can smell him from my seat, but I bite my tongue. Instead, I paste on a smile and listen to his tales, trying to make a connection I still yearn for. I listen to Howie and the twins asking polite questions, the familiar eggshells crunching beneath our feet.

Before long I feel the tendrils of exhaustion and my hope that this time will be different quietly shifts to hopes the visit will pass quickly and without incident.

It began the next day. Quietly. I could see his anger and frustration build through lunch with my parents. He shoves the table, stands up and walks away, trying to sort it out but his damaged brain is incapable of accepting anything not going his way. I know he feels trapped. He wanted to leave today to go back to Zaq but the repairs on his car are going to keep him here for one extra day. I know he is afraid of what will happen if he disappoints Zaq. It is too much for him. He begins by turning on me, his voice raising with each question.

"Why didn't you listen to me when I told you to order the parts?"

"Why can't you make them get it done faster?"

"WHAT'S WRONG WITH YOU MOTHER!?"

Experience taught me this was a losing battle. But I thought maybe, just maybe, my parents' presence would change things.

"Fin, sometimes things don't happen as fast as we'd like. It's just one more day. Let's start over."

We all held our breath. He quieted. Silently we got in the car to go shopping. I knew we were in that fragile between place. Where anything I say is ammunition and silence gives him air to reignite the smoldering fire. I try small talk.

"It's been a long time since we've all been shopping together."

That's all he needed.

"I shouldn't be here. I should be driving home. If you listened to me in the first place my car would be ready. I *told* you and *told* you to schedule the appointment. You should have known how long it would take. Oh, now you're not answering me. Wipe that fucking smile off your face, Stacy. You are so fucking stupid"

The pace of his attacks picked up and his volume increased.

It's like watching a ball of fire picking up speed and getting hotter as it barrels toward you. The best bet is to run the other way but sometimes it's impossible.

We were in a moving car. Our safety at risk; I tried to stay calm and diffuse the situation.

"Fin, I'm sorry you feel that way. You are obviously in no condition to go shopping with your grandmother."

I made a U-turn.

"Stop the car. I'm getting out!"

He reached for the door handle. I saw a school bus in my rear-view mirror and reached across to grab his arm to stop him from opening the door. He bent down like an animal and bit me. Shocked, I pulled my hand back. Somehow, I managed to pull to the curb and let him out.

At that moment I looked in the rear-view mirror and saw my mom, Fin's Nana, who had been sitting quietly in the back seat, and realized she finally understood. She had tried but had always held hope that we could change him. Now her eyes showed a sadness that wasn't there a little while ago. She had been let into a version of my life I'd held close. Up until this moment, the stories I'd shared had been carefully curated for their ears. What just transpired felt like sending a child into an X-rated movie.

I'd killed her naivete. It's impossible for anyone to understand the feelings of helplessness, anger, and sadness I experience when Fin is around.

Something in me broke. I realized I could not do this anymore.

I left Fin on the side of the road. Barely looking back, I sped off with my mom in the back seat. I squeaked out an "I'm sorry," even though we both knew none was needed, and I tried to answer her questions before they started coming.

"He won't get far. He's way too out of shape to walk all

the way. Let me drop you off at home and I'll go back. And again, I'm sorry."

Why was I sorry?

I was sorry our day of multi-generational shopping, no matter how much a pipe dream, was ruined.

I was sorry she had to see that.

I was sorry it happened—that Fin was so broken that he had become a stranger, and a seemingly dangerous one at that.

I hoped I'd spoken enough and answered her immediate questions and that she'd hold off on any others until a later date. I was lucky. We drove the short distance in silence. When I stopped in front of her condo I got out and we hugged. The sadness in her eyes was unmistakable, but I also saw reassurance that I'd done everything I could for Fin. In that moment I realized my mom and I were more in sync than ever.

I found Fin sitting outside Dunkin' Donuts about a mile from where he jumped out of the car. He got back in the car silently, but once we started driving home, he started in again. I let him rant, trying to tune him out and get us home, where we could get out of the car and I could get away from him.

I stared through the back door sliders. He was sitting on one of the Adirondack chairs surrounding the fire pit we built when we redid the backyard patio a few years earlier. Watching him slumped in the chair, smoking cigarettes, tossing one after the other into the fire pit, I noted the dirt on his feet was so deep it looked like an outline of the flip flops abandoned on the back steps, and I wondered how we got here.

My throat was raw from the yelling of the past few hours, and I was sure if I looked in the mirror, I would find a face far older than my fifty-four years. I was completely drained from the years of trying to help, guide, force, threaten, make him take care of himself. I was exhausted from bouncing between feeling so sorry for what life has dealt him, to being so angry and trapped I worried I might hurt him. It had been an uphill battle for years and while I understood I couldn't fix everything, I needed to find some peace.

I opened the back door and sat down in the smoke-filled silence.

"Fin, I can't do this anymore."

Before I could get any further, he turned to look at me with a vacant vengeance in his eyes.

"Can't do what?"

"I can't go through this with you. You are sick, and you need help. And until you get the help you need you can't stay in our house…"

He cut me off and laughed in my face.

"Oh sure, just what you and Dad always wanted. To get me out. Wash your hands of me. Then you can have your precious family with your perfect two children."

I knew he was trying to steer me off track, thrashing out with a historically surefire way to deflect and soften me. But not today. From between clenched teeth I swallowed and continued.

"You know that's not true, and I'm not going there. After your car is fixed, you will leave and hopefully get the help you need. I want nothing more than to have a relationship with you…"

More laughter, but I continued anyway.

"But you have become abusive, and I can't do it anymore. I won't."

The insults continued flying but I ignored them. I stood up to go inside and he stood up, coming close enough that I coughed from the smell of cigarettes on his breath. He was glaring at me, his hands clenched at his sides. I instinctively took a step back. He responded with a satisfied laugh as if he were trying to scare me. My hands were itching to smack him across the face but instead I just whispered.

"I'm going inside. I mean what I said. Clean up your cigarettes."

Setting boundaries was much easier than keeping them was ever going to be. Telling people became a strategy itself. Part gaining permission, and part reinforcement, each person helping build the army I needed to be sure I didn't retreat at the first sign of trouble.

After a few back-and-forth texts, I finally got Marnie on the phone. Since Fin stopped being her patient, we had maintained a friendship, mostly social, with the occasional lunch date sprinkled in. I tried to respect the change in our relationship and refrained from seeking advice.

The last time we spoke, she asked how Fin was doing, and I tried to keep it light but something in my eyes must have told her there was more than I was saying.

"He's living in Arkansas with this guy Zaq and seems to be in love. He's looking for a doctor to help him transition. He still doesn't have a job and we're still sending him money. It's up and down. Today, right now, it's okay."

"And the days it's not okay?" she asked.

I leaned forward…the warmth of my coffee long gone.

"It's hard to admit, but it's easier for me with him in Arkansas. Sometimes he seems like he's doing well, filled with promises of getting help, a job, social security, you name it. Other times, he's downright vicious. I'm at the point where I actually panic at the thought of him coming home."

I realized I had been rambling; I sat up smiling apologetically, but grateful for her friendship and her opinion.

Marnie leaned back in her chair and crossed her arms, transforming us into client/therapist once again.

"I think Fin will continue like this. Back and forth with

promises for the next few years. He is going to grow more independent, but *very* slowly. I would say by thirty you will see some real independence from him. But you should expect to support him until then."

She looked apologetic, but I was satisfied. At least I had something concrete to hold on to.

I had thought about that conversation often since then, keeping age thirty as an unwritten goal.

But now, at twenty-four, Fin was six years short, leaving me with questions. Were we forcing him into an independence he wasn't ready for? Were our reasons enough? Were we doing the right thing? I hoped she could help.

I was sitting out back in the early fall sun. Our backyard had become a haven in the past year since Covid sent us into various forms of lockdown. Late summer pink and purple flowers slowly being covered by brightly colored orange, yellow, and red leaves felt like a metaphor for how my own life was changing. I pulled two chairs to face each other, creating a makeshift lounge chair as I waited for Marnie to pick up at our agreed upon time.

Marnie's voice broke the silence, and after a few minutes of catch-up, we got down to business. I could picture her in her car, files piled on the seat next to her, each one filled with notes and backgrounds detailing children like Fin. Thankful she was giving me time even though we no longer had a file, I quickly filled her in on the details of our last visit and the conclusions Howie and I had come to.

"We told him when he was here, but our plan is to clarify it both on the phone and then in a letter. There's three parts. Part one is that he can't come to visit until he is seeing a therapist, and that therapist tells us he is safe to visit. Part two is that when and if he comes to visit again, he cannot stay in our house. We will put him up in a hotel. This is so we can both have down time and hopefully a successful visit. It will also help me feel safe and not trapped when he is here. And part three is that he has until January and then we are done supporting him. I just can't do it anymore. It's not helping motivate him to get a job or do anything. Maybe this will. I don't know if any of this will work, but what I do know is that when he is home, I realized that he can't wait to leave and honestly, I can't wait for him to leave. It makes me feel so bad. I just keep thinking that you said we are in it until thirty…"

Marnie listened and then took it further, clarifying her comments from our last meeting.

"When I said thirty, it was to give you a guide, some kind of expectations. I didn't expect him to get as deep into his illness as he has. From what you're saying now, he is very comfortable where he lives. He is surrounded by people like him. When he comes here, he feels like a failure. You and Fin live in two very different worlds and accepting that will make things easier for both of you. My bet is that this is it. He might get a little better, but the Fin you see now is the adult Fin. Thirty was a marker I gave to give him time to mature, but I think we're there."

She continued talking about adulthood and how in normal development children have a period of time after high school where they still turn to you for advice and support, and then the next time, they need less. Progressive independence she called it. Fin had not made any steps toward this, and all signs showed he wasn't going to without a push.

That made sense to me. It was something I could hold on to.

I sat in my backyard long after we hung up. I barely heard the lawn mowers crisscrossing the modest plots of lawn on my block. Marnie's words allowed me to let go of age thirty as a target and gave permission to our plan to set our first real boundary.

I just needed to know Howie agreed. I knew these boundaries were what I needed to feel safe. I knew it was a chance for Fin to become independent. And I knew it was our best chance to have a relationship. But I couldn't be in this alone for two reasons. First, there was strength in conviction, and second, if our stance had the opposite effect and Fin ended up in trouble or worse, I needed to know this was a choice we made and agreed upon together. I needed to know this for myself, for Howie, for Fin, and to be able to explain it to Emily and Leo.

I set up a meeting with Dr. Sanders. Good old Dr. Sanders. He knew our story and we could always count on him to give it to us straight.

It was still post-Covid and Dr. Sanders was not seeing patients in person yet. Howie and I sat side by side on our couch, laptop between us, waiting to be let into our Zoom appointment. We had discussed it all, reliving each painful detail of the last week endlessly, and we both agreed it was time to let go. Trying to make Fin a part of our world was like pushing a square peg into a round hole.

I felt a sense of peace as I sat on the couch with Howie, a blanket from our storage ottoman wrapped around me like a hug. I leaned on Howie's shoulder, the perfect support for my head, strong and unyielding from years of weightlifting yet warm and welcoming. I felt a kiss on the top of my head as I snuggled in. That small gesture reminded me of the bond we had. The veil of anger I had been seeing everything through seemed to have lifted and I was left with acceptance that felt more stable than anything I had felt in years.

I positioned our laptop between us and clicked on the link Dr. Sanders sent for our session. We weren't in the waiting room long before Dr. Sanders' face appeared on our screen. We said hello and adjusted our laptop so both of us appeared on the screen. I hadn't spoken to Dr. Sanders in over a year, and the pandemic seemed to have aged him as it did all of us. Maybe I was projecting as I knew I avoided my own image as much as I could.

We exchanged a few pleasantries, and then Howie began.

"Stacy and I wanted to talk to you about Fin."

He started to explain the events of the past week; I jumped in periodically and soon took over the floor completely. I had been there for all of it, and we both wanted to catch Dr. Sanders up as quickly as possible.

"And I told him he wasn't welcome here anymore until he is getting the help he needs and a therapist he is seeing regularly tells me he is safe to come back. But I don't think he can ever stay here again."

I was out of breath from reliving it; Howie finished.

"So, in addition to not letting him come back here, we've also discussed cutting him off financially. We wanted a professional to help us with this. So…go. You have forty minutes to solve this with us!"

We all laughed, glad for a moment of levity, and then Dr. Sanders began. He wasn't surprised by anything we told him given Fin's history and diagnosis. He was more amazed we hadn't made this call earlier.

"Frankly, I'm surprised you held on for as long as you did. And as long as you keep helping him, he will continue taking. You keep negotiating with him when all he is doing is manipulating you. He will say whatever it takes to get you to give him what he wants. And when he doesn't get what he wants he turns on you. This will go on for as long as you allow it, and for as long as he believes you will allow it. The only way this cycle can break is for you to break it. But you have to both be committed."

We listened as he spoke. Dr. Sanders was not a therapist that let you do all the talking. He shared stories of his own and painted pictures of what we could expect. The scenarios were real and not always easy to see, but I appreciated his candor. It helped us face reality.

"Dr. Sanders, I'm done." My voice broke, but I took a deep breath, swallowing past the lump in my throat.

"I can't do this anymore. I hate how I feel about him, but I hate when he's here. As soon as the phone rings, my stomach ties up in knots. We have discussed it is time to cut him off, but it is easy to say and harder to do. What will happen? What kind of parents do that?"

"Stacy, here's what will happen. Nothing. He will go on to find other ways to get what he wants. Maybe he will get the help he needs or maybe not. He will continue calling you, begging, even threatening, until he believes you aren't his escape or his meal ticket. Then he will stop. You may not hear from him as often, or not at all for a while. But my guess is he'll figure something out. When he does, he'll come back. His life will continue to be a series of crises, but he will stop dropping them on you as frequently or as heavily. This is just the beginning and it will be hard, but things will get easier. But if you want this to work, you have to set your boundaries and stick to them."

"That's what I'm worried about." I didn't want to throw Howie under the bus, so I said it delicately, but I had been dealing with Fin almost alone for a while now. It was a combination of my availability and the fact that Fin was still splitting us and refused to talk to Howie. Since most of our time with Fin now was crisis management, there just wasn't the down time needed to work on their relationship.

Dr. Sanders laid it out with such brutal clarity I winced at his words. We had to be prepared for Fin to end up in a homeless shelter, living in his car, in jail, or worse. He would blame us, yell, threaten, each escalating the more desperate he became. Or he could cut us off all together. Above it all, we had to stand firm and together.

I remained calm as he spoke, but the last part sent my heart racing again. I believed his lifestyle was not sustainable and there was a distinct possibility that I could end up burying my own child. I needed to know that we did everything we could to help and that I didn't make the decision that ultimately put him there alone.

Perhaps out of desperation, or perhaps Dr. Sanders' words empowered me, but I was finally able to give voice to my fears. Howie looked directly at me when I finished and pulled me in a little closer, kissing the top of my head.

"We're in this together and I am ready to do this."

We would see.

It was Thanksgiving morning. The first one I'd hosted in two years. We weren't having a big crowd, but the preparations were the same. It was a tradition we had perfected and one I cherished, even though I complained relentlessly. Maybe it was the two-year break, a European trip to visit Leo and Emily while they were studying abroad, and then a global pandemic had made gathering impossible. But I was very excited to have as many of the usual players together for the familiar meal.

Thanksgiving had always been my favorite holiday, and I carried many of the same traditions from my childhood to my table in New Jersey. Plans for our family's favorite holiday began early. My brother, Michael, and his family only came every other year; sometimes Howie's mom came up from Florida, and there had even been years I invited distant cousins on my mom's side to join us. But the die hards, the bones of our Thanksgivings since I took over the tradition many years before, had been our family, my parents, my grandmother *(until she passed away)*, and my cousin.

Jonathan and his family were unable to come up from

Richmond this year. I understood but was really missing them. At fifty-six, Jon finally had enough teaching inner city high school kids the past year. He took a retirement incentive and went back to being Jack, his alter ego from his car selling days. Back at it, Jon/Jack had to be on the lot first thing on black Friday. We hadn't seen them in two years and while we Zoomed holidays, birthdays, and even hosted a trivia night, I was looking forward to the chaos his kids, Sonny, *(16)*, Max *(13)*, Phoebe *(10)*, and Will *(7)* brought.

Instead, this year seemed uncharacteristically quiet. The twins were still sleeping upstairs. They would be down soon to stake out their spots on the sectional. I could picture it all unfolding as it had many years before. Spread out and cozily tucked in with blankets from the storage ottoman they would watch the Thanksgiving Day parade *(again after a pandemic hiatus)*, followed by the dog show. Howie would join them after showering from his morning run, and I would listen from the kitchen as I checked and basted the turkey every twenty minutes or so.

By the time they woke up, I had already set the day in motion. The smells from a stuffed turkey in the oven and cider mulling in the crockpot filled the house with memories and nostalgia from years past. I was enjoying the day. It was quieter. Perhaps a good way to again host guests in our home after the pandemic. I used to thrive on the rush of successfully pulling off a Thanksgiving—a herculean effort for normal families. Superhero status with ours. Not anymore. I knew better. I had let go.

In the quiet of the morning, I thought of the other person missing from this year's table. Fin. I acknowledged the relief and through that found I was able to miss him. From the kitchen I saw the table set for six. With my parents, there's only four of us. As I continued to stare, I saw memories from Thanksgivings past unfold like an old movie reel. Absent were the yelling, crying, and cleaning up of the messes caused by Fin's illness. My memory had made the necessary edits, and I was able to clearly see our family of five. All of us stuffed into our kitchen set up with various bowls, blenders, and ingredients following the family recipes I carefully laid out. The kids tiptoeing to the outside fridge to steal tastes of Nana's stuffing before it even went into the turkey. Their conspiratorial giggles when they were younger and believed they were hiding their mischief and later their uninhibited laughter as they rooted on their favorite picks at the dog show. Each year their eager hands dug into the appetizers, reluctantly getting off the couch to greet our guests as I yelled from the kitchen, and later all five of us snuggling back on the couch, recounting stories from the day, enjoying our food coma and plans for leftovers.

I knew I made the right decision. I knew it would be easier without him, and I was finally holding true to a boundary I set, preventing another visit like the last visit and hopefully pushing Fin toward some healing and independence. Still, I missed him.

I picked up the phone to tell him. He answered.

"Hello?"

My heart felt fuller hearing him. "Good morning, sweetie. Happy Thanksgiving."

"Hi, Mom. Happy Thanksgiving to you."

We settled into the easier conversations we had been finding as of late. Since we stopped supporting him, our phone calls weren't filled with requests for money. We had room for other topics. As we discussed our plans for the day, I addressed the elephant in the room.

"I miss you. Are you sad you can't be with us this year?"

There was a short hesitation, and it made me wonder if this was something he actually considered when we discussed him being unable to join us until he was in consistent therapy and I was told by the therapist that he would be safe to visit. Safe meaning he would not be abusive toward me or anyone else. Basically, he needed to be able to hold it together in a family situation. He had just begun online therapy, but we were not there yet.

"Not really…not because I don't want to be there with y'all, but because I am not in a place where it would be good for any of us."

I breathed a sigh of relief. I didn't have to shoulder the burden of keeping him away—we seemed to agree it was for the best. It made my next words easier.

"Well, I miss you. You are part of our family, and I hope you do the work so we can be together again soon."

He was silent. We both were. I wondered if we were both thinking about what that will look like, knowing it had to be different, but simultaneously hoping it would be the same.

I didn't want to get off yet.

As with all conversations with Fin, he jumped to the next topic, listing all the problems he was facing with Zaq. Like a slap in the face, I returned immediately to a heightened state of frustration where I am caught in his chaos. Perhaps strengthened by the connections we've been making or weakened by missing him on our special holiday, I didn't hold back.

"I don't know what to say, Fin. I can't solve all your problems anymore…"

He cut me off mid-sentence and said with a clarity and authority I had never heard before, "I don't need you to fix it, Mom. I just need you to listen. Can you do that?"

With another sigh of relief twenty years in the making, the permission I could never give myself was granted to me by my child.

I replied simply, "I can do that."

And as the turkey cooked, the twins came downstairs, and our Thanksgiving unfolded, I sat on the phone with my son, and I listened.

EPILOGUE

One of the hardest parts about writing this memoir is that I can't tie it up in a pretty bow at the end. Coping with mental illness is difficult and messy, but sharing our experiences is important. It is the only way to reduce the stigma and help each other. So while it is often far from pretty—even in that category of *you can't make this stuff up*—it is my real life and it is still going on. And that's more than okay with me.

Many of you have asked if Fin knew about me writing this book, and if so, how did he feel about it? The answer is yes, Fin knew, and he has even been part of my memory for some of the stories and timeline. I'll let him share how he felt about it all in his own words on the pages to follow. I am grateful to him for not only his support, but for many things that writing this book has helped me realize.

Thanks to you, Fin, I'm a better person.

When I started this journey as your mom, I thought I was an adult. But I didn't really know what that meant.

I thought I had it all figured out. But now I know I still don't.

I thought I knew what I wanted out of life. But now I know that sometimes the best parts of life are the ones that come disguised as the worst parts.

I thought I was one of the lucky ones. Now I know that I am.

I thought I could figure out a way to solve all the problems life handed me on my own. Now I know that the answer to solving many of those problems is turning to others.

I thought I could only be happy with the fairytale life I envisioned. Now I know that happiness is a choice and fairytales can be rewritten.

I thought liking myself depended on how others saw me. Now I know it only depends on how I see myself.

I thought I knew everything. Now I know learning never ends.

I thought finding peace was one of my many activities. Now I know it is often inactivity.

I thought I was an adult and that qualified me to be your mother. Now I know that you helped me grow up.

I thought happiness could only be achieved once all the messiness was cleaned up. Now I know it is a choice made every single day, even in the face of chaos.

I thought needing and asking for help made me weak. Now I understand knowing when to ask for help and doing so makes me strong.

I thought being an adult meant I had it all figured out. Now I know being an adult is knowing I'll never figure it all out.

I thought setting boundaries meant putting up walls to keep me safe. Now I know boundaries are so we can both grow on our own and hopefully meet somewhere in the middle.

I thought life was short so I should hurry up and get where I was going. Now I know, if I'm lucky, life is long, leaving plenty of room to take side trips, enjoy the journey, and make changes along the way.

Now, at fifty-eight, I think I can safely say I'm an adult, but I don't really know. And that's okay. It's actually exciting and liberating. I feel lighter knowing I can't control everything. The weight I carried as a twenty-eight-year-old girl working so hard to become pregnant, or a mother frantically folding laundry and putting toys away to maintain some semblance of order, or the guilt of being unable to save you from a disease, doesn't crush me like it used to. I understand the problems aren't gone, but experience has given me hindsight to know we will get through whatever is thrown at us. The shoes haven't stopped dropping, they just feel lighter; sometimes I barely hear them. Like slippers on a floor.

THROUGH FIN'S EYES

When my mom first told me about this book being published, I told her how excited I was for her. Inside I was seething. It wasn't until a week or two later that I called her back and voiced my concerns. My biggest fear was that the book was going to be a tell-all of my darkest moments. Moments that I still felt ashamed of and guilty for. She listened and stressed the level of maturity I showed in voicing my concerns, then she immediately went to work putting them to rest. I nodded along and felt slightly better. I gave the green light and supported her as she wrote, but I was still worried.

So, when she called me to ask if I would write a short passage for the book I was unsure of what to do. Part of me wanted to say I do not support the book and only support my mother as she has supported me throughout my life. Another part of me just wanted to continue the charade. Still another part of me didn't want to do anything other than curl up and cry because of everything I feared this book would be. I was angry that this was even happening.

I called my mom and asked her to read the book to make sure what I wrote was in line with what she had written. But I was lying. I thought by reading the book I would confirm it was the tell-all book of closet skeletons I feared, and I could write my piece to trash her in the way I was sure she deserved.

She agreed and told me that aside from her editor(s) I was the first person to read the book. As I began the prologue my worst fears seemed to come to light.

I started questioning myself. *Why am I really doing this? Why do I want to be angry? Who am I truly angry at?*

It was in that moment, that I finally acknowledged the answers I had known all along but didn't like: selfishness, fear, and myself.

As I looked around our home and at the beautiful family we were building, the most important questions I had never dared to ask finally came to light. *How do I want to be seen in the eyes of those who truly matter to me? Do I really want to give in and once again become the unlovable monster that my fears and shame had convinced me I am? The monster I was so sure this book would show on every page? Or do I want to be the man that they and I know myself to be? The father and husband whose heart is inevitably plastered on his sleeve no matter how many layers he may don.*

Taking one last glance around the room, my eyes lingered for a moment on the faces of the ones who matter most to me; taking a deep breath, I started again with a new perspective. Taking myself out as much as I could, I read as though it were written by and about someone else. Then I got to Chapter 3. Reading *And Baby Makes Three* changed my entire perspective and view on this book. It helped me understand so much about my history that I never knew and made me realize how much I was wanted and loved. From that point on I was fully in it. I read the rest without anger or fear in my heart. Instead, with a love and understanding that I had never allowed myself to have. And with a newfound pride in my mother.

As my mother has said time and time again, *BPD is a mean disease.* You are constantly at war with yourself. You know what you're doing and how you're reacting is wrong. You want to stop. You know you need to. But you are frozen in a loop controlled by an illness. You feel powerless. Yet you are hyper aware of how awful you are being. So much so that you end up being more angry at yourself than you ever are at the person who is the object of your anger. If you, or someone you know, loves someone with BPD, please keep all this in mind.

And for anyone out there struggling with BPD, please know you are not the monster you see yourself as. There are people out there who do love you and you deserve that love. Work on loving yourself and allowing yourself to be loved. I know that's easier said than done, but after having read this book, I now see the love that was there all along. And I now see just how much this disease, and the fear that I am unlovable was so powerful that I made it my reality.

My mother is a woman who embodies what it means to be a mother. Someone who fights for and loves her children even when they won't let her. Someone who never gives up no matter how hard it gets. She is someone who sees the good in people and finds a way to show it to them so they can see it in themselves. While it took a journey of my own to get here, I can honestly say I support and am proud of *Searching for Slippers* and my mom, and that reading it has had a tremendous impact on my life. I truly hope you find the same.

My mom once told me that if this book can help to ease the pain and struggles faced by just one family, no even just one person than she would feel fulfilled and accomplished. Congratulations Mommy, it has. It has helped me, and my family that I am now building as an adult. So that officially makes one, but I can say with certainty that mine is only the first. The first of many

I love you to the moon and stars and back again.

-Fin

ACKNOWLEDGEMENTS

I've read many books in my life, but rarely do I do more than skim the acknowledgements. After writing my own, I now understand that in many ways it is the most important part. Without the people mentioned in the acknowledgements, there would be no book, and the version of me who was able to write the preceding pages would simply not have existed.

I am so profoundly grateful to everyone who has helped me arrive at this point. Both the life I write about, and the writing of the story itself, could not have happened without all of you.

To Howie - my husband, my best friend, my rock, my biggest cheerleader, and yes, my superman. Without you there would be no me. Thank you for the fairytale. I am grateful for you and for us every single day.

To our twingles, Leo and Emily. I know it isn't easy to revisit some parts of our lives. Thank you for understanding why and supporting me through it all. For making room for me to follow a dream, for listening when I needed it, for giving advice, suggestions, and even design help. I could not be more proud to be your mom. Keep fighting for what you believe in and I believe you will change the world.

To my parents for being there throughout my life, unwaveringly, even when I pushed you away. And for learning what you needed to understand - always.

To the many other members of my family who didn't always know what we were going through, but loved us anyway.

To all my friends, whether called out by name or not. You know who you are. I could not, and would not want to, do it without you. Thank you for knowing when I needed a shoulder to cry on, a good laugh, or even a night out. Whether I see you a few times a year or a few times a week, I am thankful for you every single day. I couldn't live my life or have written about it without you.

To all our therapists and doctors. Thank you for discussing some of the finer points about treatment and Borderline Personality Disorder for the writing of this book, and more importantly, for helping us at critical points throughout our life.

To Jenn Tuma-Young and everyone at Inspired Girl Publishing Group for taking my call, talking to me, and for taking a chance on me. I will never forget your words "we publish two memoirs a year and would like you to be one of them". They are the words that changed my life. Writing a memoir is an intense and deeply personal journey, and I couldn't have done this without your guidance, understanding, and friendship.

And lastly, to Fin for making me a mom and for all that followed. Your support was the green light I needed to go ahead and write. I will always be proud of you and cheering you on as you take on life's challenges and continue to grow. Please know there is nothing that could make me want any other life than the one I have.

RESOURCES FOR READERS

For additional mental health resources, please visit the QR code below.

www.ingramcontent.com/pod-product-compliance
Lightning Source LLC
Jackson TN
JSHW021911220625
86549JS00001B/3